REFRAMING INTIMACY

REFRAMING INTIMACY

A Faith-Filled Guide to Sex, Desire, and Connection

Kelsey Mathias, OTR/L, PRPC, and Larry Mathias

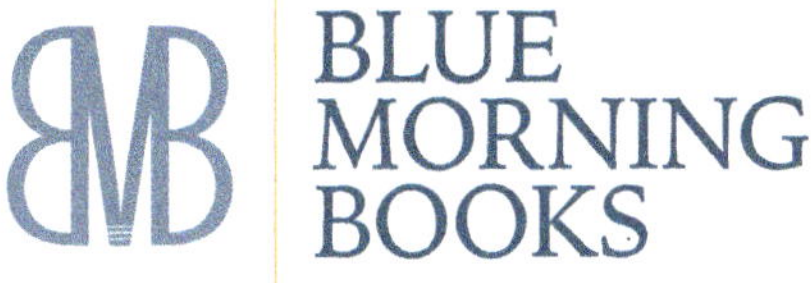

BLUE
MORNING
BOOKS

Published by Blue Morning Books
Poolesville, MD
bluemorningbooks.com

Disclaimer
This book is intended for informational and spiritual encouragement only. Readers should consult qualified healthcare providers, licensed counselors, or trusted spiritual leaders for advice regarding their specific situations. The authors and publisher make no guarantees regarding outcomes and disclaim liability for any loss, injury, or damages resulting from the application of the information contained in this book.

ISBN: 978-1-971826-01-1
Library of Congress Control Number: 2026932825

Cover and interior design by Jennifer Folden, Riverton Design Collective
Cover art by Saltoli/Adobe Stock
Composition by Manila Typesetting Company
Printing by Gasch Printing

BISAC: REL012050—RELIGION / Christian Living / Love & Marriage
SEL034000—SELF-HELP / Sexual Instruction
HEA042000—HEALTH & FITNESS / Sexuality

Printed and bound in the United States of America

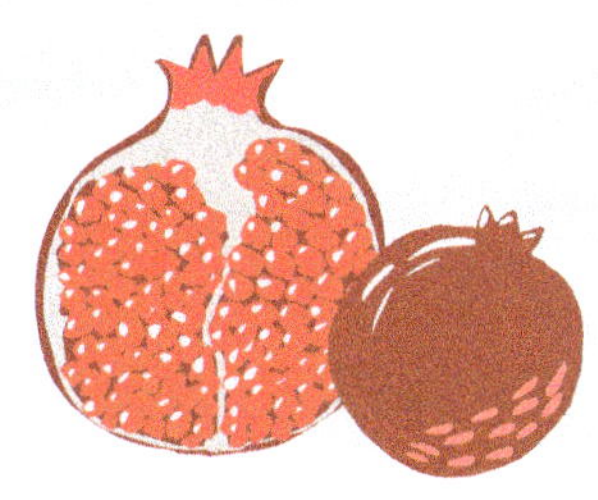

CONTENTS

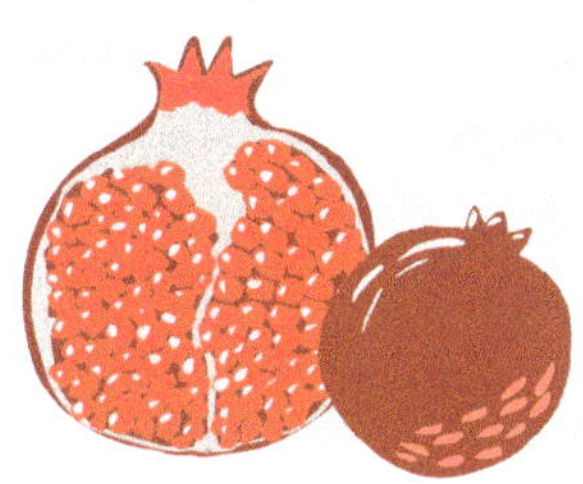

INTRODUCTION

OUR "WHY"

We—Kelsey and Larry—met almost twenty years ago at a ministry school in the Rio Grande Valley of Texas. It was intrigue at first sight. We quickly became best friends, bonding over deep conversations while mock-sparring with drink stoppers from a local coffee shop. Our shared quirkiness was paired with a united vision to impact the world for good. Our friendship grew into love. About a year later, Larry became a family ministry pastor at the same church where we had met.

When we went through premarital counseling, and we read the recommended books. They were books that inspired good conversations, but they often left us with more questions: Do men really think that way? Do women really think that way? Why is the pleasure of women secondary? How many of these stereotypes are actually helpful? We questioned whether we were "normal" or if something was wrong with us because our experiences didn't match the portrayals we had read.

If there was any sense of shame in that season, it was subtle, not overt. Larry is a confident 5'7"; Kelsey is a confident 6'1". With a six-inch height difference in the opposite direction of what society and church culture often expect, we were already accustomed to not fitting neatly into prescribed norms. As we read books that leaned heavily on narrow definitions of masculinity, femininity, and desire, we felt less personally attacked and more perplexed. We wondered whether the authors had all consulted the same small group of people to arrive at their conclusions of how men and women operate. They overlooked the wide range of bodies, relationships, and expressions that exist within God's creation.

There were moments, especially for Kelsey, when the question quietly surfaced: Do I need to change who I am to fit this picture? Again and again, we returned to Scripture and recognized that many of the books we were reading reflected cultural opinion rather than biblical truth. What helped us move forward was the growing clarity that different doesn't equate with deficiency. God's design allows for far more variation than many of these resources suggested.

While Larry continued in pastoral ministry, we moved to Colorado, where Kelsey became an occupational therapist specializing in pelvic health. She became a rehabilitation expert for all things related to bladder, bowel, and sexual function and sex counseling. In her clinical work, a consistent pattern emerged: Many clients, male and female, described frustrations that echoed themes we had already noticed in our own reading and conversations with clinicians and ministers. At the same time, Larry was encountering many of these same struggles in pastoral counseling, as couples wrestled with shame, misunderstanding, and rigid expectations around intimacy. The Christian resources they used often weren't relatable, rarely addressed physical intimacy in meaningful ways, lacked an evidence-based foundation, and sometimes even caused harm. Couples sought ways to build intimacy without shame or pain and to talk about these sensitive topics in ways that fostered connection rather than division.

Now, we are working to flip the script. By combining Larry's biblical training and fifteen years of experience in family ministry and pastoral counseling with Kelsey's clinical sexual health specialization, this guide provides education that is relatable, shame-free, evidence-based, and rooted in God's design. We address the whole person—mind, body, and soul—because healthy intimacy is not just about techniques or biology, but about connection, purpose, and wholeness in marriage. If this sounds like what you are looking for, you've opened the right book!

THE BIG PICTURE

We believe that God created intimacy as a gift for marriage—not just for procreation or physical release, but for deep connection that reflects His covenant love. That's why our approach integrates three dimensions:

- *Mind:* understanding your own and your spouse's mental and emotional wiring
- *Body:* honoring the physical realities that influence pleasure, comfort, and desire
- *Soul:* seeing intimacy as a sacred, spiritual bond that mirrors God's love for His people

These three dimensions don't stand alone. They are like a root system beneath the soil. When one root is parched, the others begin to wilt. Sometimes a sickness in one area migrates into another. The opposite is also true; healing in one area is just as contagious. Nourishment in one root eventually feeds every branch.

THE STORIES YOU'LL READ

The stories you'll read here come from years of working with couples—listening, learning, and noticing the patterns that show up repeatedly. They are true to the kinds of experiences so many people have shared with us, but they don't belong to any one person. We've blended details and changed names to honor the privacy of every client and couple while still capturing the heart of what real people have lived.

Consider Maya, a new mom in her early postpartum months. Her story shows how stress in one area of life can affect other areas of the mind, body, and soul. After having her baby, she feels self-conscious about the physical changes in her body which begins to shape her thoughts. She questions her attractiveness and wonders whether intimacy will ever be the same again. As her mind grows more guarded, her desire to connect feels low. Physically, she withdraws from intimacy and activities that previously gave her joy—like hiking or date nights—because being in her body feels vulnerable. That loss of adventure and the inability to see herself as she was before motherhood leaves Maya's soul longing for meaning and purpose beyond diapers and feedings. One vulnerable area can profoundly affect other areas.

The good news is that this interconnectedness works the other way too. When one area is nourished, eventually every area gets fed. One couple asked God to help them see intimacy not as pressure or performance but as part of their worship. They also asked God to show them the good things in each other they had been overlooking. That spiritual step (soul) softened some mild resentment that was starting to build. Their communication became more tender (mind) and, almost surprisingly to them, their desire for one another physically (body) increased.

One husband committed to taking evening walks with his wife, just to help her feel cared for and heard. That physical act of presence made her feel emotionally safe (mind), which opened her heart to spiritual connection (soul) and renewed desire (body) for him.

The couples in this guide share a mutual desire to pursue God and deepen intimacy with one another—and deep, connected intimacy takes time. We hear you: You want a timeline! For some, deep changes can happen in days. More realistically, it can take weeks, months, and years of dedicated connection. Intimacy deepens over time and ebbs and flows through life's seasons. Basically, developing intimacy takes the time that it takes.

Remember, intimacy is never just physical, or just emotional, or just spiritual. It's all three! The mind, body, and soul work together in harmony. Our approach doesn't separate these dimensions but invites couples to see how tending to one area can bring life to the others. Our work is grounded in both Scripture and science, honoring God's Word while drawing from reliable, evidence-based research in sexual health.

HOW TO USE THIS GUIDE

We won't tell you there's one right way to have a healthy sex life or shame you for what you don't know or for what you've struggled with. Instead, we celebrate what's already good, gently address what can be improved, and remind you that your worth and identity are rooted in Christ, not performance.

Set the Space

This guide is designed for you and your spouse to use as a couple. If you read it on your own and then talk about it with your spouse, that works too. If you are working through it simultaneously, find a quiet, comfortable space: no phones, no kids, and no distractions. Give your full attention to each other. Intimacy conversations are the most productive when you feel unrushed and present.

This guide is set up in three main parts:

- **Part 1. Getting on the Same Page** goes through the basics of sex and intimacy. It covers the things you wish that Mom, Dad, school, and the church (or someone you trusted) would have told you, but no one did—or they did something, but it wasn't what you needed.
- **Part 2. Ten Conversations Every Couple Needs to Have about Sex and Intimacy** is where you get to practice (easy, tiger, not *that* kind of practice— yet) ten guided talks that may include laughter, eyerolls, and maybe a little blushing.
- **Part 3. Putting Intimacy into Practice** is the section that some of you might skip to as soon as you crack the book open. We get it. It's where we encourage you to get hands-on (and maybe clothes-off) and try some things in the bedroom that you may have never tried before—and that's a lot of fun (no judgement here). However, we strongly encourage you to at least read Part 1 and do a couple of the discussions from Part 2 first.

Once you have engaged in a couple of discussions from Part 2, it's alright to take a little bit of a choose-your-own-sex-adventure approach, alternating between Parts 2 and 3. You may want to proceed in the exact order in which this guide is written. That's also fine! What matters most is that you and your spouse get on the same page about what intimacy looks like for you. By the time you get to the end of this guide, our hope is that you and your spouse will connect in mind, body, and soul.

One Conversation at a Time

Don't try to tackle the entire guide in one sitting. We see you: highlighters out, powered by cold brew and holy zeal—and maybe some horniness. Rushing intimacy is like microwaving a steak: technically possible, but highly regrettable. After reading Part 1, aim for one discussion per week or every other week. Maybe throw in something from Part 3. Make a plan that fits your schedule, and don't be afraid to take your time as you work through this guide. Many of us may feel that, if we just try harder and do more, then things will get better; however, tenderness, patience, and humility are needed when working on developing intimacy. If you find yourself trying to push through the guide to be done and for things to get better, remind yourself that, instead of trying harder, do as author and mental health therapist Aundi Kolber has coined and "try softer.[1]"

Healing

Healing is a process that takes time. As you work through this guide, you may uncover wounds and the results of trauma that have been ingrained in your body, mind, and soul. Do not shy away from these feelings—embrace your humanity. This guide may also bring to light needs, emotions, or patterns that extend beyond the scope of what this text can address on its own, and that's okay. If this is the case, a licensed mental health care provider can be a great resource. One place where you can find help is at www.psychologytoday.com, where you can also filter to find Christian-based providers, if preferred.

In moments of panic, fear, and disconnection, our prayer for you is that the words of our Savior echo through your soul: "Come to me, all you who are weary and burdened, and I will give you rest. Take my yoke upon you and learn from me, for I am gentle and humble in heart, and you will find rest for your souls. For my yoke is easy and my burden is light" (Matthew 11:28–30).

Pray Together First

Each time you sit down to talk through this guide, consider praying together. Ask the Holy Spirit to guide your words, to guard your hearts, and to help you hear each other with grace. Prayer shifts the atmosphere from defensiveness to openness.

MARRIAGE IS NOT A LICENSE TO HARM

Everything in this guide is written for marriages that are safe, mutual, and life giving. Intimacy flourishes when both husband and wife feel honored, heard, and free to say "no" (or "not yet") without fear of anger, manipulation, silence, or any kind of harm.

If any of the following feel true for you right now, please pause and reach out for help now. Sexual abuse—and abuse in general—happens in far too many marriages. You are worth safety, dignity, and care, and God hates the abuse of His daughters and sons. Get help now if:

- You're afraid to say no or to set a boundary.
- Touch (even non-sexual) often feels demanding or punishing.
- Past or present coercion, force, or any non-consensual act has happened.
- You feel chronically small, guilty, or responsible for your spouse's emotions around sex.

You are not alone, and healing is possible. Start with a trusted pastor, licensed counselor, or call the National Domestic Violence Hotline (800-799-7233) or text "START" to 88788. When safety and mutual delight exist, the conversations, reflections, and intimacy-building exercises in this guide can be a source of beautiful connection. Until then, your well-being matters more than any exercise in this guide. Please seek out any help you need.

CHECK YOUR MINDSET

As you step into the conversations in this guide, remember: This process is not a performance review! It's an invitation to understand and be understood. Come with curiosity instead of judgment and assume the best of each other, even if you hear something surprising or hard.

This guide will help you uncover what already works well in your relationship, discover new ways to connect, and learn how to navigate the more difficult or delicate areas of intimacy. There will be moments when you feel affirmed, and moments that might stretch you. Stretching is part of growth.

FORCING THE ISSUE ISN'T FIXING THE ISSUE

If you feel tension rising between you and your spouse during discussions, pause and return later rather than pushing through. It's better to resume when you're both calm than it is to force a conversation when emotions are high. Forcing your way through conflict rarely builds intimacy; it usually just builds volume levels.

Most importantly, remember that you are not broken. You are learning how to love as Jesus loves. God didn't design intimacy as a set of rigid rules that can be broken with one misstep, but as a joyful, lifelong journey toward deeper connection. The kind of intimacy you will learn in this guide is about moving toward, not away from, each other.

Ephesians 4:2–3 reminds us to "be completely humble and gentle; be patient, bearing with one another in love. Make every effort to keep the unity of the Spirit through the bond of peace." In other words, approach each conversation with humility (not with "I'm right, and you should just see it!"), gentleness (stop the "you always" or "you never" phrases), patience (resist thoughts such as "why is this still a struggle?"), and determined unity.

As you pray, reflect, and show up for each other, remember power exists not only in grace and honesty but also in a well-timed joke and the unity that comes from loving as God first loved you.

OPENING PRAYER FOR INTIMACY CONVERSATIONS

Father, thank You for the gift of our marriage and the ways You've brought us together. We invite You into this moment. Help us to speak truth with love, to listen with grace, and to understand each other's hearts. Remind us that we are on the same team, and that our love is rooted in Your love for us. Give us courage where we need to be honest; gentleness where we need to be tender; and joy in discovering more about one another. May this conversation draw us closer to each other and to You. Amen.

---

[1]Kolber, Aundi. *Try Softer: A Fresh Approach to Move Us Out of Anxiety, Stress, and Survival Mode—and into a Life of Connection and Joy*. Carol Stream, IL: Tyndale House Publishers, 2020.

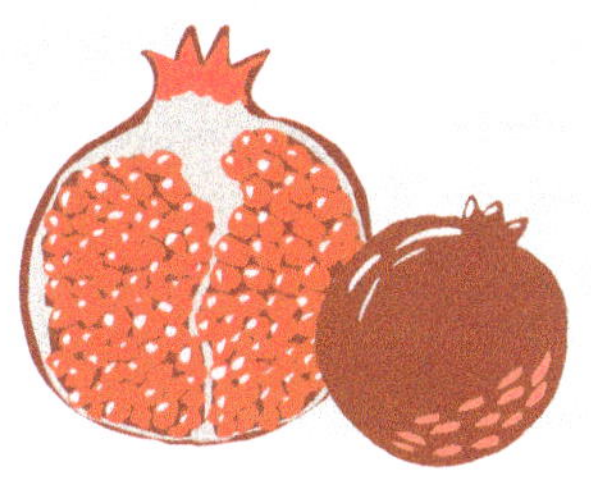

PART 1.

Getting on the Same Page

HIGHLIGHTS

female anatomy • male anatomy • how male and female anatomy overlap • Gas and Brakes Checklist • Connected Intimacy Check-In

---

Many of us grew up with little accurate teaching about sexual anatomy. Some of what we learned came from playground rumors, health class gloss-overs, or church settings that avoided the topic of anatomy altogether. Larry was home-schooled and went the extra mile: He skipped the reproductive anatomy chapter entirely because he thought, I'm never getting married, so why would I ever need to know that?

Bless his heart—poor ninth-grade Larry.

Every part of the body you've been given by God deserves to be known, respected, and cared for. Learning about anatomy is not dirty or inappropriate. It's part of taking care of God's creation. *You* are part of God's creation. Understanding your spouse's body and your own is an act of love, a way to care for the person God entrusted to you. Learning the body parts and how they function lets your brain and body know what is going on, reduces anxiety, and makes way for better communication. It also helps couples work together to address any challenges with desire, arousal, or satisfaction that may come up while going through this guide.

God's design for intimacy involves complex and beautiful anatomy in both men and women. If you've ever stared at an anatomy diagram as Michael Scott from *The Office* did when he was faced with a spreadsheet—confused, concerned, and about to declare bankruptcy—you are among friends.

Let's break it down.

FEMALE ANATOMY

The **vulva** includes the **outer labia** (*labia majora*) and **inner labia** (*labia minora*), which protect sensitive structures and can swell with arousal. The **clitoris** (it does exist and is not a mythological creature), with over eight thousand nerve endings, is the primary organ for sexual pleasure. It has an external **glans** (the external part of the clitoris that is often most sensitive to touch) and a larger internal structure extending alongside the vaginal walls. The **vestibule** is the sensitive tissue around the vaginal opening that leads into the vaginal canal (a muscular, flexible passage that also plays a role in childbirth). The **Bartholin's glands**, located inside the vestibule, are two pea-sized structures that produce lubrication. Inside, the cervix connects the vagina to the uterus. The pelvic floor muscles support the internal organs, influence sensation, and can tighten or relax during arousal.

Male and female erectile tissue all starts from the same original blueprint but shows up differently on the outside. In men, erections are easy to spot. In women, most of the erectile tissue is tucked under the surface, so you only see the glans clitoris and clitoral hood externally. In other words, both men and women experience erections. One is just a lot more obvious at first glance. Check out Figure 1 and Figure 2 for a visual of female sexual anatomy. Figure 3 shows how female anatomy becomes erect during arousal.

Figure 1. External and internal female sexual anatomy illustrating the relationship between visible structures and the larger internal components.

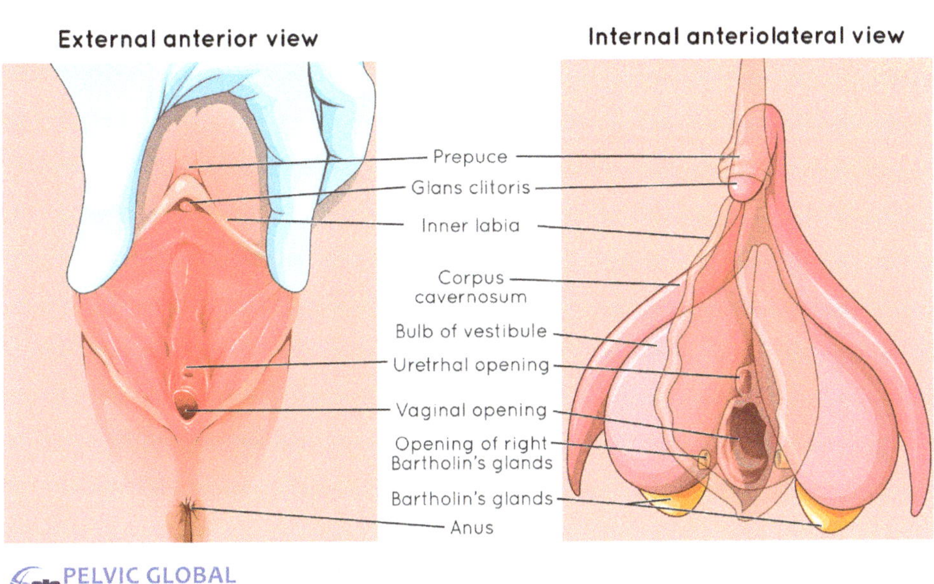

Note. Used with permission from Pelvic Guru®, LLC, as a Pelvic Global Member.

Figure 2. External female genital anatomy: visible structures of the vulva.

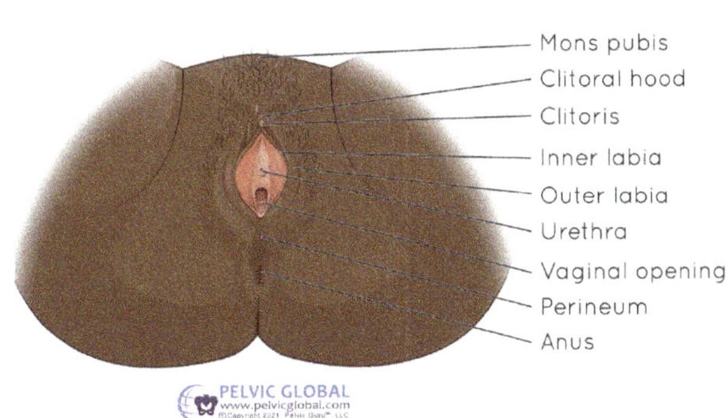

Note. Used with permission from Pelvic Guru®, LLC, as a Pelvic Global Member.

Figure 3. Changes in female sexual anatomy during arousal, comparing the clitoris at rest and during arousal.

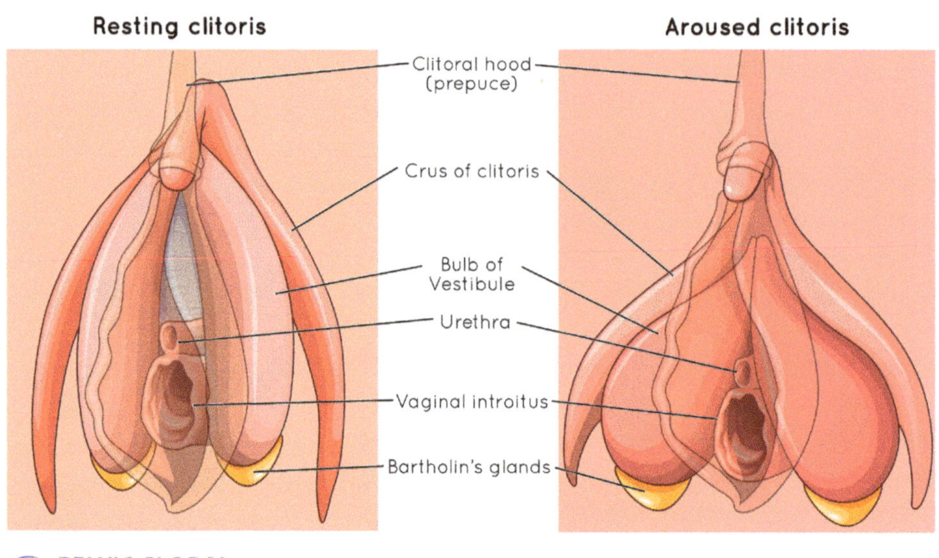

Note. Used with permission from Pelvic Guru®, LLC, as a Pelvic Global Member.

What Happens During Female Physical Arousal?

In Figures 1–3, you can see where the clitoris lines up with female external anatomy. Here is what happens during physical arousal and excitement:

- **Clitoris and labia minora:** Increased blood flow to the clitoris occurs. The clitoris becomes swollen and engorged.
- **Bulbs of the vestibule:** Increased blood flow causes tissue to become erect and can cause enhanced sensitivity to the area.
- **Vagina:** Increased blood flow can increase sensation. The inner portion of the vagina, close to the cervix, gets longer and wider to accommodate penetration.
- **Pelvic floor muscles:** These muscles tighten and support clitoral erections and pleasurable sensations. They also play a key role in orgasm.

- **Lubrication is produced:** The vaginal walls, Bartholin's glands, and cervical mucus all contribute to lubrication to minimize friction and increase comfort and pleasure. The production of natural lubrication is very sensitive to hormones, stress, hydration, and medications. Using over-the-counter lubrication can be helpful—using lube isn't cheating the system; it's being smart. We will dive more into lube later in the chapter.

The Female Sexual Response Cycle

Sexual response is not linear for many women. Desire, arousal, and satisfaction don't always happen in a straight line. For many women, feelings of desire might come after they start to feel physically aroused or even after a connection with a partner. This is called **responsive desire**. For some, desire may occur spontaneously. Both responses are normal, and the overall cycle more closely resembles a loop where emotions, physical sensations, and closeness all play a role, and they can happen in any order.[1] An orgasm occurs during the emotional and physical satisfaction phase. This cycle reflects the beautiful complexity God built into our bodies and relationships and is an incredible reminder that intimacy is dynamic and relational, not formulaic.

Let's dive deeper into what's at play.

Emotional Intimacy

Emotional intimacy is feeling deeply connected, seen, valued, and safe with your spouse. It creates a space for your interior world to become known—your secret fears, biggest dreams, and the things that make you feel embarrassed or proud—and to be held with tender trust by your spouse. This kind of trust and vulnerability says, "I can show you the deepest parts of me that no one else knows because I believe you would not use it against me." Such trust and closeness make vulnerability feel inviting rather than terrifying. It will feel like "I'm safe and loved" instead of "Oh no! Panic! Retreat!" For many women, emotional connection and intimacy greatly influence how their bodies respond to physical intimacy. Deep, emotional connection can shape desire, arousal, and the ability to enter physical closeness.

Romans 12:10 encourages us to "be devoted to one another in love. Honor one another above yourselves." This verse invites couples to actively honor and cherish each other, creating a safe space where trust grows and connection happens.

Tim and Anne Evans of Real Life Ministries capture the essence of this verse beautifully. Anne shares,

> Our marriage grew deeper when we learned to listen to each other. As co-leaders, we had to come together as a team like Adam and Eve in the garden, we needed to take equal responsibility since we equally had a relationship with the Lord and each other. It's in those ongoing conversations, filled with grace and patience, that each of us felt truly valued and safe. Creating that environment of emotional safety is key; it's where honest intimacy starts and flourishes.[2]

Sometimes emotional intimacy looks like surviving the what's-wrong dance. You know the one! One spouse asks, "What's wrong?" The other insists, "Nothing," and a mysteriously repeated two-step of suspicion and reassurance begins. The good news? With enough laughter and grace, that dance can eventually turn into a confident waltz of honesty.

To grow emotional intimacy, try nightly rituals, such as sharing one small appreciation or asking fun how-was-your-day questions. Emotional intimacy is less about perfection and more about showing up, mess and all.

Sexual Activators in an Appropriate Context

Sexual activators—in an appropriate context—are anything that tells your brain, Hey, this is actually a great moment for intimacy. Sometimes it's a flirty look—and sometimes it's a dishwasher that someone else loaded. Context is everything. The same gesture that feels magical on a date night can feel overwhelming when a toddler is shrieking through the baby monitor.

Scripture reminds us, "Daughters of Jerusalem, I charge you . . . Do not arouse or awaken love until it so desires" (Song of Solomon 2:7). This verse captures the importance of waiting for the right time and conditions for intimacy. Let love and desire bloom naturally, rather than hurrying or forcing it.

Spontaneous Desire

Spontaneous desire occurs when desire for intimacy comes out of nowhere, with no specific trigger. It's the surprise party of the desire world—awesome when it happens, but no one should expect it to happen every weekend.

Again, Song of Solomon has some great descriptions of spontaneous desire. Pretty much all of Chapter 7 can be summed up in Verse 10: "I belong to my beloved, and his desire is for me." After this verse, the bride invites the groom in and shows similar desire. This is a poetic celebration of mutual longing and delight. It captures how desire sometimes erupts spontaneously, a natural overflow of love and belonging.

Biological, Social, and Psychological Factors

Your sexual response isn't just one system. Things happening in us and around us let us know whether we are ready for sex.

- **Biological:** Hormones, health, sleep, nervous system (and whether your body says, Yes! or says, Try again later)
- **Social:** How your relationship is going, cultural or church messages about sex, privacy (Is the door locked?)
- **Psychological:** Stress level, body confidence, mental health (Is your brain still replaying that awkward comment from earlier?)

Some days everything lines up just right, and your mind, body, and relationship feel connected and ready for intimacy. Other days, not so much: Stress, disconnection, or exhaustion can make desire feel far away or slow to start.

The good news is that change is possible. With curiosity, communication, and a bit of patience, couples can learn what supports desire and what shuts it down. Together, you can move toward more connection, pleasure, and confidence.

Sexual Arousal

Sexual arousal is the physical part of turning on: increased sensitivity in the genitals and surrounding tissues, lubrication, blood flow, and your body saying, If we keep going, this is going to be fun, but here's the important part: arousal is a green light, not a contract. You can feel physically turned on and still not want sex at that moment. Both your brain and your body get a say—and you're allowed to change your mind anytime with no justification required. No one, not even your spouse, should insist you keep going just because you began the journey.

The Bible puts it this way: "The wife does not have authority over her own body but yields it to her husband. In the same way, the husband does not have authority over his own body but yields it to his wife" (1 Corinthians 7:4). This verse has often been misused and misread to pressure women into sex as an obligation or duty. That interpretation misses the heart of this passage entirely.

"Yielding" does not mean you lose your right to say no but quite the opposite. It means that your body is so precious to your spouse that he or she will never force, pressure, or demand something of you that goes beyond your boundaries. Wives, because your husband has yielded to you, he chooses to honor your boundaries over his own wants and desires. He yields to your "no" or your "not right now," and you yield to his "no," because you both value each other's hearts more than you value a physical act. Mutual belonging means both partners get a voice and a veto. Sex is a shared dance, not a solo performance under obligation.

THE DEATH OF DUTY SEX

If you use 1 Corinthians 7:4 to pressure your spouse, you are not "yielding" to them; you are quite literally taking from them. True authority in marriage is the power to protect your spouse, not to exert your power over them in order to use them. When sex becomes something done out of obligation rather than mutual desire, it is linked with lower relationship satisfaction, particularly for women.[3]

Duty sex does not strengthen intimacy. It trains your body and mind to associate sex with stress rather than connection. This kind of pressure dishonors your spouse and the One whose very image they bear.

Desire and arousal often go hand in hand in a complementary fashion, but they are different from one another.

- Desire equals wanting.
- Arousal equals your body responding.

Either desire or arousal can show up first, and they can swap which one is in charge at any moment. A woman can have increased vaginal lubrication and not desire sex until the social and psychological factors line up. She can also desire sex during at a part of her menstrual cycle when she has decreased vaginal lubrication, and she can enhance her biological factors by using a store-bought lubricant. Both desire and arousal are normal. Both desire and arousal are good.

Emotional and Physical Satisfaction

Emotional and physical satisfaction is that we-are-in-a-good-place feeling after intimacy. It's when the body and heart both exhale. It can look like orgasm,

A NOTE ON LUBE

Lubricant (lube) is a product that adds moisture and glide to reduce friction during sexual activity. It helps reduce friction and increase comfort so your body can relax and enjoy the moment. It supports pleasure, protects delicate tissue, and helps intimacy feel good for both partners instead of rushed or painful. Lube can help make intimacy more satisfying for both spouses by honoring your body's needs in real time.

A marriage has many reasons for when using lube is not only helpful but wise. You might find yourself reaching for it more often during times of stress, after childbirth, during that latter half of the menstrual cycle, during perimenopause or postmenopause, or simply when your body needs a little extra moisture. Some couples prefer to always use lube. That's totally normal.

We've heard misconceptions such as, "As the husband, I should be enough for her, so she shouldn't need it." Some people worry using lube is unbiblical because they believe sex should happen naturally without any outside help, or they think needing it means something is spiritually wrong in the marriage. These concerns often come from cultural or church messages rather than Scripture. Using lube does not conflict with a biblical view of intimacy. Tools that support comfort, pleasure, and loving connection are consistent with caring for one another in marriage. Needing or wanting to use lube is not a commentary on a wife's desire or arousal for her husband. It simply reflects that our bodies and our seasons change, and we get to care for them with wisdom.

TYPES OF LUBE AND WHEN TO USE THEM

- **Water-based lubes** are the most versatile. You can safely use them with both latex and non-latex condoms, and with most vibrators. They clean up easily, though you may need to reapply more often.

- **Silicone-based** lubes feel slicker and last longer. They are safe with condoms, but if you are using a silicone toy you might want to check if the lube is compatible because some silicone formulas may wear the toy's surface.

- **Oil-based lubes** (natural oils or petroleum-based) feel very slick and last a long time. They should not be used with latex condoms because they can weaken the barrier. They also may be incompatible with certain vibrator materials, may shift pH or increase irritation risk, and can stain fabric.

INGREDIENTS TO AVOID

- Avoid glycerin or sugar-based additives. They can increase risk of yeast infections or skin irritation.

- Avoid lubes with fragrances, dyes, or flavor additives. They can increase risk of yeast infections or skin irritation.

- Avoid using cooking oils, petroleum jelly, or generic body lotions as lubricants. They are not typically designed for sexual use, may degrade condoms or toys, and may alter tissue pH.

SUMMARY

Lube is a practical tool for comfort, pleasure, and safety. Pick the right type for the situation. Read the label. If something stings, changes color, or causes discomfort, then stop, rinse, and switch. Your use of lube does not mean you are less attracted or less intimate. It means you're prioritizing comfort and connection.

closeness, laughter, relief, or simply snuggling and knowing you're on the same team. It's about the entire connection, not just one moment at the end.

What does an orgasm feel like for a woman? An orgasm for a woman is a reflexive release of sexual tension that happens when the nervous system, body, and mind are sufficiently aroused and feel safe. Physically, it often includes rhythmic contractions of the pelvic floor muscles and uterus, along with a wave of pleasurable sensation that can be localized in the genitals or experienced more broadly throughout the body. Yes, an orgasm can literally make your toes curl. Emotionally, it may feel like a sense of release, warmth, closeness, or deep relaxation. Orgasms do not feel the same for every woman or even the same for the same woman every time. Some orgasms are intense and obvious. Others are subtle, spreading, or quiet. Some orgasms feel primarily physical, while others feel more emotional or relational.

Emotional satisfaction means feeling safe, valued, and deeply connected, while physical satisfaction involves the sense of comfort and fulfillment that comes from mutual touch and presence. From a nervous system perspective, these are not separate experiences. Emotional safety tells the brain that connection is safe, allowing the body to shift into arousal, pleasure, and responsiveness. When the body gets the signal from the brain that it is safe and open to pleasurable experiences, the body is able to feel all of the delights and joys of being intimate with your spouse. When emotional or physical safety is missing, often because of stress, fatigue, or pain, the nervous system prioritizes protection over connection. That protective response can interrupt desire, arousal, or orgasm. Together, emotional and physical satisfaction form the foundation of a satisfying intimate relationship.

Research shows that emotional and physical intimacy are intertwined and essential for a healthy marriage, fostering mutual trust, respect, and lasting connection.[4] When both are present, partners experience greater overall satisfaction and resilience in their relationship. See Figure 4 for a visual of the female sexual response cycle.

Figure 4. The female sexual response cycle.

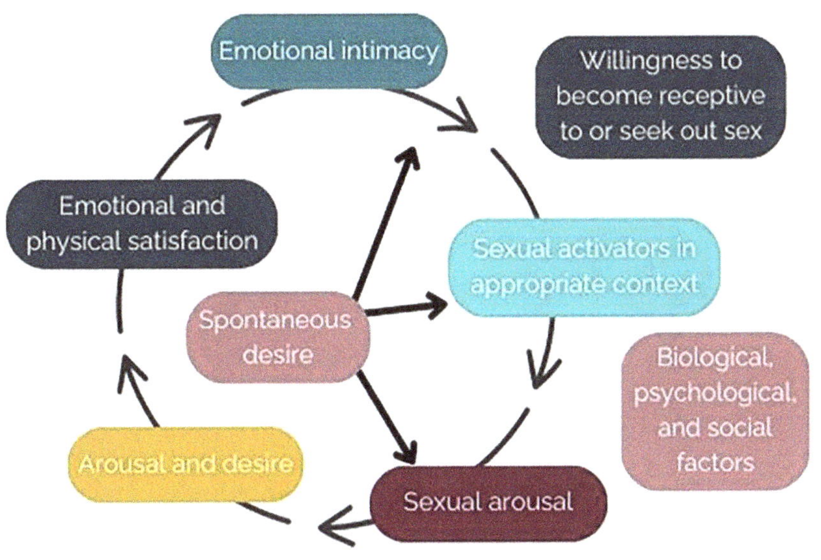

WHAT IS NORMAL AND WHEN TO CHECK IN

Women's sexual response can change day to day and season to season. Shifts in desire, arousal, and satisfaction are common. Stress, hormones, sleep, body image, connection with a spouse, and the mental load of life all influence how the body and mind respond to intimacy. Variability is normal.

It can be helpful to talk with a health care provider or pelvic health occupational or physical therapist if any of the following show up:

- Pain before, during, or after sexual activity
- Ongoing difficulty with arousal or orgasm that causes frustration or worry
- Persistent low desire that feels very different from your normal
- Leaking urine, pelvic pressure, or other changes in pelvic function at any point or time
- Concern or fear related to intimacy after childbirth, trauma, or medical procedures

Reaching out for support is a wise and courageous step that shows care for your body and your marriage. Healthy intimacy grows when both physical needs and emotional needs are honored.

There is nothing wrong with you for needing help. You deserve to feel comfortable, confident, and connected.

MALE ANATOMY

The **penis** includes the **shaft** and **glans** (tip), which is rich in nerve endings for pleasure. In uncircumcised men, the **foreskin** is a fold of skin that covers the glans and also contains sensitive nerve endings that contribute to sexual sensation. The erectile tissue fills with blood during arousal, causing an erection. The **scrotum** houses the **testicles,** which produce sperm and testosterone. The **prostate gland,** located internally, contributes to seminal fluid and can also be a source of pleasurable sensation.

What Happens During Male Physical Arousal

Check out Figure 5 to see the primary structures involved in male sexual function. It's important to note that arousal can look different from one experience

Figure 5. External anatomy of an uncircumcised penis (a) and a circumcised penis (b), illustrating key structures involved in sensation and function.

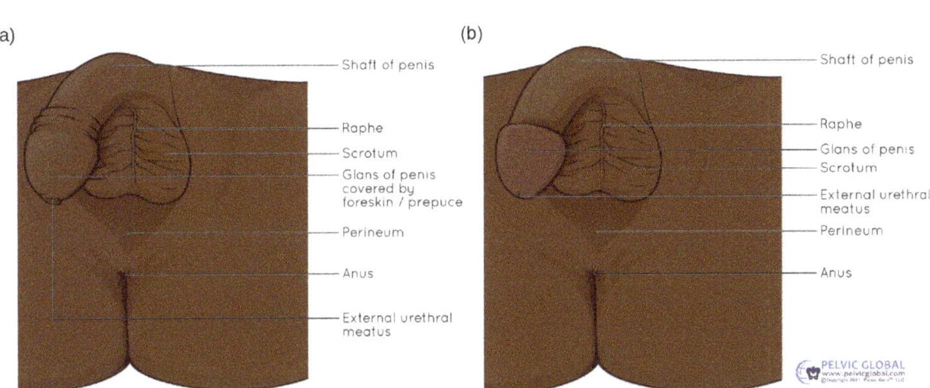

Note. Used with permission from Pelvic Guru®, LLC, as a Pelvic Global Member.

to the next. Erections can be more or less firm, may take more or less time, and can change during intimacy. Needing more stimulation or different stimulation is common and normal. Supplements like lubrication, different positions, or changes in pace are not cheats or crutches. They are tools that help intimacy feel good for both partners.

Here is what happens in the body during physical arousal:

- **Penis:** Increased blood flow fills the erectile tissue inside the penis. It becomes firm and enlarged so penetration can be comfortable and possible. Sensitivity increases during this time.
- **Scrotum and testicles:** The scrotum tightens and lifts the testicles slightly toward the body. Temperature regulation matters here because sperm production prefers a cooler environment. Some men notice changes more than others.
- **Pelvic floor muscle:** These muscles tighten and support erections and pleasurable sensations. They also play a key role in orgasm.
- **Pre-ejaculate fluid:** Small glands near the urethra release a clear fluid. This helps neutralize the environment in the urethra and can add some lubrication. Pre-ejaculate can contain sperm, so it is important to note that the pull-out method is not a reliable form of contraception.

- **Breathing and heart rate:** Breathing may become faster and more shallow. Heart rate increases as the nervous system shifts into a state of excitement.

The Male Sexual Response Cycle

The male sexual response cycle is more complex than "erection equals ready." What you see isn't always what you get. Because the penis is outside the body, it's easy to assume an erection is the only sign that a man is ready for sex—but there's a lot more going on under the hood (or under the sweatpants).

Here's a more complete picture of male sexual response, based on physiology and recent research.

Desire

That I-want-to-be-close-to-you feeling shows mental interest or curiosity about intimacy. Sometimes desire arises spontaneously without a clear trigger, and other times you have to intentionally shift focus before the desire kicks in. Studies highlight that men's sexual desire is more variable than once thought, with different patterns and intensities depending on a variety of factors.[5]

Arousal

Physiologically, blood flow increases, the penis gets firm (an erection), breathing and heart rate pick up, and muscle tension builds. Pre-ejaculate fluid might make an appearance. The body is thinking, "This could be fun, should we keep going?"

Orgasm

Muscles around the penis contract rhythmically, pleasure peaks, and the brain fires off a confetti cannon of happy chemicals. This may or may not include ejaculation. This may confuse some, but orgasm and ejaculation are close cousins, not identical twins. Orgasm is the experience of pleasure. Ejaculation is the release of fluid. They often happen together, but they are controlled by different processes in the body. When they do not line up perfectly, your body is still operating normally.

The difference between orgasm and ejaculation shows up in a few ways. For example, someone can have an orgasm without ejaculation, or ejaculation without feeling the full pleasurable peak. Both situations are common and do not mean there is a problem with the body or with intimacy. Differences in orgasms reflect the way in which the nervous system and reproductive system can respond differently in different moments.

Resolution

Resolution is the cool-down phase: relaxation, satisfaction, maybe sudden hunger—you may even need a nap. Bodies differ on their exact reaction for resolution.

Variability Is Normal (Yes, Really)

Life affects sexual response for everyone. Yes, men, too. That tough meeting at work, the baby's sleep regression, or worry over Dad's cancer diagnosis can affect the ability to have an erection. Connection, stress, sleep, anxiety, illness, medications, and emotional well-being can all influence each part of the sexual response cycle. A man can

- have an erection without wanting sex,
- want sex but struggle with arousal,
- need more time (or less) than last week, or
- orgasm earlier or later than hoped. (*Note.* Orgasming quickly often happen for those who have never experienced sex before. Give it a few weeks to build up—well—stamina.)

None of this is failure. It's just being human.

A shift in desire or arousal is almost never a reflection of a spouse's attractiveness or value. Bodies simply respond to the environment they are in. Couples talking about these changes with curiosity instead of pressure can build trust and help them work together toward intimacy that feels safe and satisfying for both people.

HOW MALE AND FEMALE ANATOMY OVERLAP

Arousal involves increased blood flow, muscle engagement, and nerve activation. Touch, emotional connection, and mental focus can all play a role. That means intimacy is always a whole-person experience, not just a mechanical act.

Similar Parts: Penis and Clitoris

When we started developing as embryos, we all started with the same body parts. As the embryo matures, the same parts develop into either the penis or the clitoris.

WHEN VARIABILITY IS NORMAL AND WHEN TO CHECK IN

Bodies do not behave the exact same way every time during sex. A change in timing or intensity or whether orgasm and ejaculation happen together is usually nothing to worry about. Men are allowed to have off days and off moments. This is part of being human, not a sign of decline or disaster.

It can be helpful to talk with a health care provider if any of the following show up:

- The change is frequent or long-lasting.
- Orgasm and ejaculation (or lack thereof) causes stress, embarrassment, or avoidance of intimacy.
- There is pain or discomfort.
- There has been a recent medical procedure.
- There are concerns while trying to conceive.

Reaching out for support does not mean failure. You are simply paying attention to your health and your connection with your spouse.

Figure 6 shows which parts started from the same tissue. If you read above and saw some overlapping functions of the penis and the clitoris, you weren't wrong! In many ways they are the same parts, organized in different ways. Isn't God cool that way?

Why Desire and Arousal Don't Always Align

The sexual response cycle doesn't always follow a straight path. It's like driving a car with a gas pedal (things that turn you on) and brake (things that turn you off). If you step on the gas but something else presses hard on the brakes, you can feel frustrated and less likely to want sex. To feel more desire, you might need to figure out what's hitting the brakes, and deal with that first, so your brain and body can respond to what excites you.[6] Knowing what hits your gas and what hits your brakes can be hard if you have never thought of your desire in this way before. Don't worry, we are here to help. We created the Gas and Brakes Checklists to help you name what fuels your desire and what might be hitting the brakes for you.

Figure 6. Comparison of the clitoris and penis structures that develop from the same embryonic tissues during fetal development.

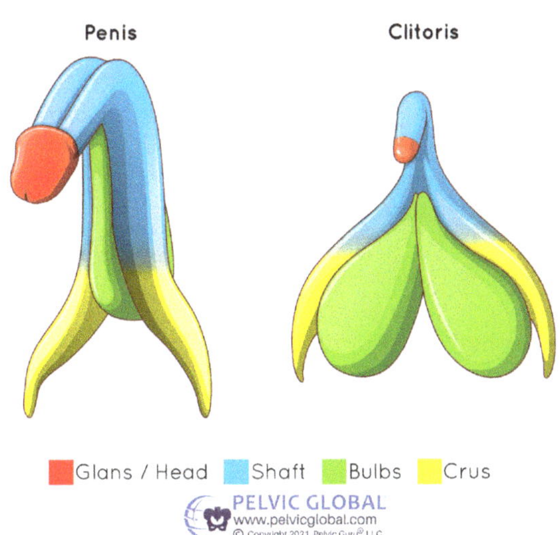

Note. Used with permission from Pelvic Guru®, LLC, as a Pelvic Global Member.

The Gas and Brakes Checklist is a tool to help you notice patterns of what turns you on and what turns you off. You can complete the checklist on your own, with your spouse, and at different seasons of life. (We've included the checklists twice so both you and your spouse can go through them separately, if desired.) What turns you on today may look different next year or even next month, and that's normal. For example, before kids, you may love feeling desired and pursued. When you have kids, this feeling may change. Having toddlers hanging on you all day long may make being wanted, pursued, or chased feel more like one more person is vying for attention. Returning to this checklist from time to time can be valuable for helping you recognize that things that have changed.

Begin by noticing what stands out rather than checking all of the boxes. Check the boxes that feel consistently true for you at this season. These checklists are intended to help give you language to understand yourself and to help facilitate gentle, compassionate, and curious conversations between you and your spouse. It can feel less intimidating to have a conversation about sex when we ask, "What's been pressing the brakes for you lately?" instead of, "Why don't you want sex?"

Those questions set very different tones to a conversation. The goal is not to force an increase in desire, but to understand what your body and nervous system respond to so that intimacy can grow.

Ready? Let's find out what's hitting your gas and what's hitting your brakes.

Gas Pedal Checklist 1

Intimacy feels inviting or appealing for me when—

Biological/physical

☐ I feel healthy and rested
☐ I experience touch that feels good to me
☐ I feel that my hormones are supporting desire right now
☐ I am enjoying certain smells, sights, or tastes
☐ I feel comfortable in my body (no pain, dryness, tension)
☐ Other ____

Social/relational

☐ I've had quality time with my spouse
☐ I feel pursued or desired
☐ I feel support through acts of service (think clean kitchen)
☐ I have space and privacy (no tiny humans wandering in)
☐ I feel seen and appreciated
☐ Other ____

Psychological/emotional

☐ I feel that my stress is manageable enough to focus on connection
☐ I feel calm and safe with you
☐ I am experiencing laughter and playfulness
☐ I feel confident and engaged in my body
☐ I feel as if we're on the same team today
☐ Other ____

Brake Pedal Checklist 1

Intimacy feels hard or unappealing for me when—

Biological/physical

☐ I am experiencing pain, discomfort, or dryness
☐ I feel exhausted or unwell
☐ I feel less desire when my spouse has body odor or poor hygiene
☐ I am taking medications that affect desire or arousal
☐ I feel as if my hormones are making desire harder to access right now
☐ I don't feel comfortable in my body right now
☐ Other ________________________

Social/relational

☐ I am carrying unresolved conflict or feeling disconnected
☐ I am dealing with interruptions or noise (kids, pets, text messages)
☐ I feel rushed or pressured
☐ I feel unseen, unappreciated, or misunderstood
☐ I am feeling tension about chores or daily life responsibilities
☐ Other ________________________

Psychological/emotional

☐ I am experiencing stress, anxiety, or mental overload
☐ I am experiencing shame or insecurity
☐ I'm worried about performance or expectations
☐ I feel emotionally distant
☐ I am too mentally overloaded to feel present in my body
☐ Other ________________________

Brakes aren't failures; they're signals. When you notice them, you can address the underlying need together. You can do everything under the sun to turn your partner on, but if they are stressed, feeling rushed, or experiencing illness, it may be hard to want sex.

Gas Pedal Checklist 2

Intimacy feels inviting or appealing for me when—

Biological/physical

☐ I feel healthy and rested
☐ I experience touch that feels good to me
☐ I feel that my hormones are supporting desire right now
☐ I am enjoying certain smells, sights, or tastes
☐ I feel comfortable in my body (no pain, dryness, tension)
☐ Other ____

Social/relational

☐ I've had quality time with my spouse
☐ I feel pursued or desired
☐ I feel support through acts of service (think clean kitchen)
☐ I have space and privacy (no tiny humans wandering in)
☐ I feel seen and appreciated
☐ Other ____

Psychological /emotional

☐ I feel that my stress is manageable enough to focus on connection
☐ I feel calm and safe with you
☐ I am experiencing laughter and playfulness
☐ I feel confident and engaged in my body
☐ I feel as if we're on the same team today
☐ Other ____

Brake Pedal Checklist 2

Intimacy feels hard or unappealing for me when—

Biological/physical

☐ I am experiencing pain, discomfort, or dryness
☐ I feel exhausted or unwell
☐ I feel less desire when my spouse has body odor or poor hygiene
☐ I am taking medications that affect desire or arousal
☐ I feel as if my hormones are making desire harder to access right now
☐ I don't feel comfortable in my body right now
☐ Other ____

Social/relational

☐ I am carrying unresolved conflict or feeling disconnected
☐ I am dealing with interruptions or noise (kids, pets, text messages)
☐ I feel rushed or pressured
☐ I feel unseen, unappreciated, or misunderstood
☐ I am feeling tension about chores or daily life responsibilities
☐ Other ____

Psychological/emotional

☐ I am experiencing stress, anxiety, or mental overload
☐ I am experiencing shame or insecurity
☐ I'm worried about performance or expectations
☐ I feel emotionally distant
☐ I am too mentally overloaded to feel present in my body
☐ Other ____

Brakes aren't failures; they're signals. When you notice them, you can address the underlying need together. You can do everything under the sun to turn your partner on, but if they are stressed, feeling rushed, or experiencing illness, it may be hard to want sex.

AN IMPORTANT NOTE ON HYGIENE

Your hygiene (or lack thereof) can be hitting the brakes. Desire is highly sensory. Smell, taste, touch, and even what your brain anticipates all play a role in arousal. When hygiene is off, it can quietly slam the brakes on desire, not because someone is too picky, but because the nervous system reads unpleasant sensory input as a signal to pull back.

Good hygiene isn't about perfection or being overly polished. It's about care, consideration, and creating an environment where connection feels safe and inviting rather than distracting.

A few simple bedroom hygiene basics:

- Wash the external genital area thoroughly, including skin folds and hair-bearing areas, using mild soap and water.

- For vulvas: gentle unscented soap is fine on the outside, but never inside the vagina. The vagina is self-cleaning, and soap inside can actually cause irritation and pH imbalance.

- Dry well. Moisture can lead to odor and irritation faster than you think.

- Breath matters. Brushing teeth or a quick rinse before intimacy can make a bigger difference than you might expect.

- Fresh underwear and clean sheets matter more than fancy cologne.

- When in doubt, a quick rinse of your body before intimacy can go a long way.

Hygiene isn't about criticism or control. It's about helping your partner's body stay on the gas pedal instead of hitting the brakes.

The Elephant in the Room

Let's say none of these areas we've just discussed are problematic. Let's say the issue is something that may feel more embarrassing to talk about. What should we do or say if our partner is just not good at sex? When we get this question, the real issues are poor communication and not understanding one's body or one's spouse's body—so what do you do about it?

First, don't criticize one another. We don't know what we don't know. Many people were never taught how arousal works and how desire can vary from day to day. For example, if you or your spouse believes you have to have sex every seventy-two hours because of bad church teachings rooted in inaccurate and misused evidence, sex is likely to be less than ideal.

In other cases, disappointing sex is not about beliefs but about missing skills. Many people were never taught the skills to build pleasurable, connected sex, such as how to read a spouse's cues, how to touch in ways that increase comfort and desire, how to communicate about what feels good, or how everyday words and actions outside the bedroom shape the intimacy experienced inside it.

The good news is that you and your spouse can learn these skills. That knowledge gap, which so often contributes to disappointing or frustrating sex, is exactly what this book is here to address.

We recommend working through every part of this guide. Knowing how your bodies work and then working through the ten discussions in Part 2 will get you a long way. Then you'll come to Part 3, "Putting Intimacy into Practice." That gives both of you the chance to develop the practical skills needed for unforgettable moments in the bedroom. If you continue to struggle after working through this book, we highly recommend sex counseling which allows a professional to help you with your and your spouse's specific needs.

Can We Talk a Little More about Orgasms?

Orgasms are for everyone, but not everyone regularly—or sometimes ever—experiences orgasms. Studies tell us that while roughly ninety-five of men orgasm during a sexual encounter, only sixty-five percent of women do.[7] That, our friends, is commonly referred to as the "orgasm gap." Imagine if about four out of ten women told their husbands, "Hey, you aren't going to experience orgasm during sex tonight—or maybe ever again. I just don't think you need to orgasm for this to be a good experience for us." We think this is something husbands would take issue with—and we think it's an issue that a gap in orgasm frequency exists for wives.

Fortunately, we have good evidence on how to help close this gap:

- **Educate yourself.** Learn about anatomy and pleasure.

- **Focus on foreplay.** It takes men an average of five to seven minutes to orgasm. It takes women an average of thirteen to twenty minutes. More foreplay can be the game changer you need.
- **Remember the clitoris.** Don't go straight for it, but most women require some clitoral attention.
- **Use open communication.** Communicate with your spouse in a compassionately curious, non-judgmental way.

And guess what? We cover these four things in this guide. We've already knocked out education on anatomy. Part 2 focuses on facilitating open communication, and Part 3 gives plenty of practical advice on foreplay—including that oh-so-needed attention the clitoris deserves. Before moving on to Part 2 and Part 3, let's do a check-in to see where you and your spouse are.

WHY "SHE GOES FIRST" CAN HELP (AND WHEN IT DOESN'T)

Among heterosexual couples, men report "usually/always" orgasming far more often than women (about ninety-five percent for men versus sixty-five percent for women), a well-documented "orgasm gap."[8] One simple way many couples narrow that gap is by having the wife climax first. Here's why it can help:

- *It targets what most women's bodies actually need.* In a U.S. probability sample, only about eighteen percent of women said intercourse alone was enough for orgasm; about thirty-seven percent said clitoral stimulation was necessary during intercourse, and another roughly thirty-six percent said that clitoral stimulation enhanced their orgasms.[9]

- *It leverages physiology.* Arousal increases genital blood flow and lubrication, clitoral and vulvar engorgement, and typically heightens sensation and comfort for both partners. When she's already engorged and lubricated, penetration often feels better and more connected for both partners.[10,11]

A gentle caveat

If "she must go first" starts to feel like a test, arousal can begin to be blocked because of this new pressure. Treat this approach as a flexible rhythm, not a rule. Communicate, experiment, and give yourselves permission to pivot on any given day.[12]

Practical ways to put this into practice (customizing to her cues)

- **Indirect first, direct later:** Start by applying gentle pressure from fingertips or a vibrator on a low intensity over the clitoral hood (not directly on the glans), then progress as comfort rises.

- **Patterns and pressure:** With a fingertip, try making slow circles, side-to-side sweeps, or up-down strokes with steady, moderate pressure, adjusting based on her feedback.

- **Dual stimulation:** Combine manual or oral clitoral stimulation with penetrative touch later in the arc, when she's already highly aroused.

- **Positions that add clitoral contact:** For example, try a woman-on-top position with gentle rocking or "grinding" so the clitoris and clitoral hood contact the pubic mound.

- **External vibrator:** Consider an external vibrator as a tool, not a crutch. Small, low-to-medium intensity devices can reliably stimulate the clitoris and are associated (population-level data) with positive sexual function and minimal adverse effects.[13]

"She goes first" isn't about "performing" a sequence (guys, this isn't the Konami Code—although she may enjoy it if you give her the ol' up, up, down, down, left, right, left, right, B, A, Start). You're trying to honor how her body was designed to respond so that both of you feel more satisfied and connected.[14,15]

CONNECTED INTIMACY CHECK-IN

Purpose

The Connected Intimacy Check-In is not a test of how good your marriage or sex life is. It is a snapshot of connection, safety, and understanding in this season of your relationship. Most of us were never taught how intimacy works in our minds, bodies, and souls, but we were often expected to figure it out once we were married.

This reflection helps you notice what feels strong, what feels sensitive or vulnerable, and where growth may be needed, without shame or pressure. This check-in occurs twice: Here, toward the beginning of this book, and again at the end. It doesn't measure perfection but aims to help you notice what has shifted as you gain language, skills, and shared understanding. Intimacy grows through awareness, curiosity, and practice, and this check-in helps your growth in intimacy.

As you move through this check-in, remember that noticing areas of struggle does not mean you—or your marriage—is failing. It means you are paying attention. God is not surprised by the places that feel confusing, tender, or heavy. Growth often begins with awareness and humility, not perfection. This check-in is not here to expose shortcomings but to gently illuminate where care, curiosity, and support may be needed. You are not behind. You are not broken. You are beloved image-bearers learning how to love one another more fully, with wisdom and grace.

This check-in looks at intimacy through five key categories that reflect how connection really grows and where couples most often get stuck. Intimacy is never just physical or just emotional or just spiritual; it is the integration of mind, body, and soul, lived out over time in a real relationship, and these categories reflect this. Together, these five areas give a fuller picture of what supports intimacy and what may be quietly blocking it.

- **Safety and being on the same team:** reflects whether both spouses feel emotionally safe, valued, and united in approaching intimacy as partners rather than opponents
- **Talking about intimacy with skill and grace:** reflects whether you have the language, boundaries, and communication skills needed to talk about sex honestly and compassionately without fear, pressure, or avoidance
- **Desire, arousal, and honoring the body:** reflects how well you understand and respond to how desire and arousal actually work in your bodies, including the impact of stress, health, seasons of life, and physical well-being
- **Integrating mind, body, and soul:** reflects whether faith and values support intimacy with freedom and meaning or whether shame, fear, or mixed messages are still shaping your experience

- **Connected intimacy and growth over time:** reflects your ability to recover from missteps, adapt across seasons, and approach intimacy as a lifelong journey of learning and connection.

Together, these categories help you see not just whether intimacy is happening but what is helping it flourish and what may need care, conversation, or support as you move forward.

Instructions

This check-in is included twice, once for each spouse. Complete your own version individually before discussing it together. Answer based on how things feel right now, not how you wish they felt or how they used to feel.

Rate each statement using the following scale:

0 Not true at all

1 Rarely true

2 Sometimes true

3 Often true

4 Very true

There are no right or wrong answers. You're obtaining information, not getting a grade.

Check-In 1

Category 1. Safety and being on the same team

1. I feel emotionally safe bringing up concerns about intimacy with my spouse.
2. I believe my spouse wants to understand my experience, even when it differs from his or hers.
3. We approach intimacy challenges as a shared issue rather than blaming one another.
4. I feel valued and cared for by my spouse outside of sexual moments.
5. When intimacy feels difficult, I trust we are still on the same team.

Category 2. Talking about intimacy with skill and grace

6. I have language to describe what I enjoy, do not enjoy, or feel unsure about sexually.
7. I feel able to say "no," "not right now," or "I need something different" without fear of consequences.

8. I feel comfortable initiating intimacy in ways that feel authentic to me.

9. We check in about intimacy rather than assuming the other person should know what we want.

10. Conversations about sex feel more curious than tense or avoidant.

Category 3. Desire, arousal, and honoring the body

11. I understand that desire does not always appear spontaneously and that this is normal.

12. I can identify personal factors that increase my openness to intimacy.

13. I can identify personal factors that decrease my openness to intimacy.

14. Physical factors such as stress, fatigue, pain, hormones, or health are acknowledged when we talk about intimacy.

15. Our approach to intimacy adapts to our bodies and seasons of life.

Category 4. Integrating mind, body, and soul

16. My faith feels integrated with intimacy rather than in conflict with it.

17. I believe pleasure and connection in marriage are good, meaningful, and something we both experience.

18. Shame does not dominate how I think about sex, my body, or my desires.

19. I feel free to bring my whole self into intimacy without fear or performance pressure.

20. Our shared values around intimacy feel life-giving rather than restrictive.

Category 5. Connected intimacy and growth over time

21. When intimacy does not go as planned, we are able to have a shame-free conversation about it and reconnect.

22. We can talk about disappointment or unmet expectations without withdrawing.

23. I feel hopeful that our intimacy can grow and change over time.

24. We approach intimacy as something we learn and practice, not something we should already know.

25. Intimacy feels like a shared journey rather than a problem to solve.

How to Score

- Rather than adding up all twenty-five questions, you will score each section separately. This helps you see where connection feels strong and where more attention may be helpful, without collapsing everything into a single number.
- Each section has five questions. Add your ratings for those five questions to get a section score.
- Each section score will fall between 0 and 20.

How to Interpret

Use the same interpretation scale for every section.

16–20

This area is currently a strength. It does not mean it is perfect, but it is likely supporting intimacy rather than blocking it. Maintain what is working and use it to support growth in other areas.

11–15

This area has a foundation with some tender spots. You may notice inconsistency or specific situations in which connection feels harder. Focus on the conversations and practices in the book that address this section.

6–10

This area likely needs attention with intent. Challenges here may be contributing to frustration, avoidance, or misunderstanding. This is a good place to slow down, to be curious, and to prioritize learning and practice. Outside help may be an option to consider.

0–5

This area feels strained or unsafe right now. This does not mean intimacy is broken or hopeless. Unresolved pain, unmet needs, or missing support may need to be addressed—perhaps by a professional. Extra care, patience, and outside help may be important here.

Reflection Questions
Answer these reflection questions on your own before discussing them together.

Which statements felt hardest to answer honestly?

____

____

____

Which areas feel most connected right now?

____

____

____

Which areas feel tender, confusing, or underdeveloped?

____

____

____

What do I hope changes as we move through this guide?

____

____

____

Check-In 2

Rate each statement using the following scale:
    0 Not true at all
    1 Rarely true
    2 Sometimes true
    3 Often true
    4 Very true

Category 1. Safety and being on the same team

6. I feel emotionally safe bringing up concerns about intimacy with my spouse.
7. I believe my spouse wants to understand my experience, even when it differs from his or hers.
8. We approach intimacy challenges as a shared issue rather than blaming one another.
9. I feel valued and cared for by my spouse outside of sexual moments.
10. When intimacy feels difficult, I trust we are still on the same team.

Category 2. Talking about intimacy with skill and grace

11. I have language to describe what I enjoy, do not enjoy, or feel unsure about sexually.
12. I feel able to say "no," "not right now," or "I need something different" without fear of consequences.
13. I feel comfortable initiating intimacy in ways that feel authentic to me.
14. We check in about intimacy rather than assuming the other person should know what we want.
15. Conversations about sex feel more curious than tense or avoidant.

Category 3. Desire, arousal, and honoring the body

16. I understand that desire does not always appear spontaneously and that this is normal.
17. I can identify personal factors that increase my openness to intimacy.
18. I can identify personal factors that decrease my openness to intimacy.
19. Physical factors such as stress, fatigue, pain, hormones, or health are acknowledged when we talk about intimacy.
20. Our approach to intimacy adapts to our bodies and seasons of life.

Category 4. Integrating mind, body, and soul

21. My faith feels integrated with intimacy rather than in conflict with it.
22. I believe pleasure and connection in marriage are good, meaningful, and something we both experience.

23. Shame does not dominate how I think about sex, my body, or my desires.
24. I feel free to bring my whole self into intimacy without fear or performance pressure.
25. Our shared values around intimacy feel life-giving rather than restrictive.

Category 5. Connected intimacy and growth over time

26. When intimacy does not go as planned, we are able to have a shame-free conversation about it and reconnect.
27. We can talk about disappointment or unmet expectations without withdrawing.
28. I feel hopeful that our intimacy can grow and change over time.
29. We approach intimacy as something we learn and practice, not something we should already know.
30. Intimacy feels like a shared journey rather than a problem to solve.

How to Score

- Rather than adding up all twenty-five questions, you will score each section separately. This helps you see where connection feels strong and where more attention may be helpful, without collapsing everything into a single number.
- Each section has five questions. Add your ratings for those five questions to get a section score.
- Each section score will fall between 0 and 20.

How to Interpret

Use the same interpretation scale for every section.

16–20

This area is currently a strength. It does not mean it is perfect, but it is likely supporting intimacy rather than blocking it. Maintain what is working and use it to support growth in other areas.

11–15

This area has a foundation with some tender spots. You may notice inconsistency or specific situations in which connection feels harder. Focus on the conversations and practices in the book that address this section.

6–10

This area likely needs attention with intent. Challenges here may be contributing to frustration, avoidance, or misunderstanding. This is a good place to slow down, to be curious, and to prioritize learning and practice. Outside help may be an option to consider.

0–5

This area feels strained or unsafe right now. This does not mean intimacy is broken or hopeless. Unresolved pain, unmet needs, or missing support may need to be addressed—perhaps by a professional. Extra care, patience, and outside help may be important here.

Reflection Questions

Answer these reflection questions on your own before discussing them together.

Which statements felt hardest to answer honestly?

____

____

____

Which areas feel most connected right now?

____

____

____

Which areas feel tender, confusing, or underdeveloped?

____

____

____

What do I hope changes as we move through this guide?

____

____

____

When This Check-In Suggests You May Need More Support

For many couples, working through these pages together will bring meaningful growth and renewed connection. For some, this check-in may also reveal that additional support would be helpful alongside the work you are doing here. Reaching out for help is not a failure of faith or effort. It is often a wise and courageous next step.

You may benefit from outside support if you notice any of the following:

- One or both of you feel unsafe saying no, setting boundaries, or expressing needs without consequences.
- There are ongoing sexual pain, physical discomfort, erectile concerns, or pelvic symptoms that do not improve with education and communication alone.
- Past sexual trauma, betrayal, or coercion is significantly impacting your ability to feel present or safe in intimacy.
- Conversations about intimacy consistently escalate into fear, anger, shutdown, or emotional withdrawal.
- Shame, anxiety, or performance pressure feel overwhelming or persistent.
- Desire has been consistently low or absent in a way that feels distressing and unexplained.
- Conflict or resentment feels stuck, and reconnection does not seem possible on your own.

These signs do not mean connected intimacy is impossible. They simply indicate that more personalized care may be needed. Helpful resources include the following:

- A licensed mental health therapist or counselor can help with communication breakdowns, anxiety, trauma, resentment, and emotional safety.
- A sex therapist (a licensed mental health therapist with additional training specific to sex and intimacy) or a sex counselor (a medical provider like an

occupational or physical therapist with additional training on sex and intimacy) can support desire differences, shame, performance pressure, and healing from past sexual wounds.

- A pelvic health occupational or physical therapist can address pain, pelvic floor dysfunction, postpartum changes, erectile concerns, and other physical barriers to intimacy.
- A medical doctor, physician assistant, nurse practitioner, or certified nurse midwife who has additional training on hormones and sexual health can help with medical tests and recommendations related to medical reasons for sexual dysfunction.
- A trusted pastor or spiritual director can help integrate faith and intimacy in life-giving ways.

If you are experiencing emotional, physical, or sexual abuse, please pause and seek help immediately. You deserve safety and care. In the United States, the National Domestic Violence Hotline is available at 800-799-7233 or by texting START to 88788.

Whether this check-in affirms your strengths, highlights areas for growth, or points you toward additional support, the goal remains the same: connection, healing, and intimacy that reflect God's love and care for both of you. Growth happens step by step, conversation by conversation, and often with help along the way. You are not meant to walk this journey alone.

1 Rosemary Basson, "A Model of Women's Sexual Arousal," *Journal of Sex & Marital Therapy* 28, no. 1 (2002): 3.

2 BibleProject, "*The Sermon on the Mount.*" YouTube video, 9:47. Uploaded January 23, 2020.

3 Jessica Sawatsky, Ryan Lindenbach, Sarah W. Gregoire, and Kyle Gregoire, "Sanctified Sexism: Effects of Purity Culture Tropes on White Christian Women's Marital and Sexual Satisfaction and Experience of Sexual Pain," Sociology of Religion 86, no. 4 (2025): 519.

4 Hyojin Yoo, Suzanne Bartle Haring, Randal D. Day, and Ramesh Gangamma, "Couple Communication, Emotional and Sexual Intimacy, and Relationship Satisfaction," *Journal of Sex & Marital Therapy* 40, no. 4 (2014): 275.

5 Dean M. Busby et al., "Challenging the Standard Model of Sexual Response: Evidence of a Variable Male Sexual Response Cycle," *Journal of Sex Research* 57, no. 7 (2019): 848.

6 Basson, "A Model of Women's Sexual Arousal," 3.

7 David A. Frederick, H. Kate St. John, Justin R. Garcia, and Elisabeth A. Lloyd, "Differences in Orgasm Frequency among Gay, Lesbian, Bisexual, and Heterosexual Men and Women in a U.S. National Sample," *Archives of Sexual Behavior* 47, no. 1 (2018): 273.

8 *Ibid.*

9 Debra Herbenick et al., "Women's Experiences with Genital Touching, Sexual Pleasure, and Orgasm: Results from a U.S. Probability Sample of Women Ages 18 to 94," *Journal of Sex & Marital Therapy* 44, no. 2 (2018): 201.

10 Tamara L. Woodard and Michael P. Diamond, "Physiologic Measures of Sexual Function in Women: A Review," *Fertility and Sterility* 92, no. 1 (2009): 19–34.

11 Kazem M. Azadzoi and Mike B. Siroky, "Neurologic Factors in Female Sexual Function and Dysfunction," *Korean Journal of Urology* 51, no. 7 (2010): 445.

12 Debra Herbenick et al., "Women's Experiences," 201.

13 Debra Herbenick et al., "Prevalence and Characteristics of Vibrator Use by Women in the United States: Results from a Nationally Representative Study," *Journal of Sexual Medicine* 6, no. 7 (2009): 1857.

14 Frederick et al., "Differences in Orgasm Frequency," 273.

15 Herbenick et al., "Women's Experiences," 201.

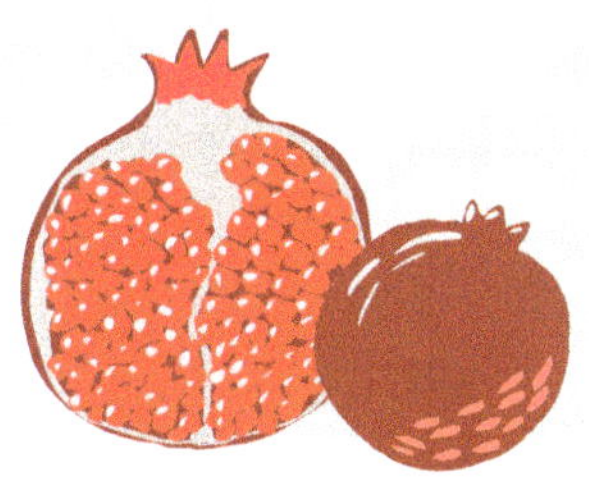

PART 2.

Ten Conversations Every Couple Needs to Have about Sex and Intimacy

HIGHLIGHTS

communication breakdowns • desire differences • body image and shame • stress, fatigue, and mental load • performance pressure • physical pain and dysfunction • resentment and unresolved conflict • healing from past sexual wounds • faith and intimacy integration • long-term spark

Understanding the beautiful design of our bodies is just the starting point of developing intimacy. God crafted us as whole beings, mind, body, and soul; therefore, intimacy is never just physical. It's woven from our thoughts, emotions, beliefs, habits, and spiritual connection. Now that we've looked at how our bodies are wonderfully made, we can turn our attention to the conversations that help us nurture that design in our marriages.

The discussions that follow are meant to guide you and your spouse through some of the most common challenges couples face in building thriving, connected intimacy. Each one blends biblical truth, evidence-based insight, and practical application, so you're not just talking about intimacy but actively strengthening it.

These conversations are not quizzes or performance reviews. They're spaces for you to grow together. Go slowly and be curious, both about your own thoughts and reactions and about your spouse's perspective. Remember that your goal is connection, not winning an argument. Approach each discussion with an open mind, a willingness to listen, and a posture of grace. It can also be helpful to schedule these discussions in advance and put that commitment on your calendars so they don't get pushed aside by the busyness of daily life. Choose a time when you're both relaxed and unlikely to be interrupted.

Read the section together, then work through the discussion questions one at a time. You don't have to finish everything in one sitting. Sometimes, the most meaningful progress comes from pausing, reflecting, and returning later. When you feel tension rising, it's not a sign of failure! You are doing the deep work of understanding one another. Maybe you reach a discussion, and it doesn't seem to fit your circumstances for this stage of life. That's fine, too. You can move on to the next discussion.

Note that when you have these discussions, a natural byproduct may be, well, having more sex. There is something about vulnerable discussions that can make us more, ahem, horny. That's great! You can always jump from one of the discussions to one of the practical exercises for the bedroom in Part 3. Your journey through this guide may become a little bit of a choose-your-own-adventure, if you will—and if one or both of you don't feel increased desire after a discussion, that's fine too. What matters most is that you walk away from these discussions feeling seen, heard, and more connected to the person that you love the most. Feel free to end each discussion by praying together and asking God to guide you in applying what you've learned in your marriage.

Discussion 1. Communication Breakdowns
- Why do we struggle to talk about intimacy?
- How can we create safety in these conversations?

Discussion 2. Desire Differences
- What's the difference between spontaneous and responsive desire?
- How can we work with mismatched frequency without misunderstanding or rejection?

Discussion 3. Body Image and Shame
- How does shame affect intimacy?
- How can we cultivate gratitude for our bodies?

Discussion 4. Stress, Fatigue, and Mental Load
- How do daily pressures affect desire and connection?

Discussion 5. Performance Pressure
- How does the pressure to "do it right" interfere with intimacy?
- How can we reclaim connection over performance?

Discussion 6. Physical Pain and Dysfunction
- How can couples compassionately address pelvic pain, erectile dysfunction, and other physical challenges using evidence-based solutions?

Discussion 7. Resentment and Unresolved Conflict
- How does lingering tension erode intimacy?
- What helps rebuild trust and emotional closeness?

Discussion 8. Healing from Past Sexual Wounds
- How do trauma, betrayal, or unhealthy past teaching shape intimacy, and what supports healing?

Discussion 9. Faith and Intimacy Integration
- What does God's holistic vision for sexual connection look like in marriage?

Discussion 10. Long-Term Spark
- How can couples keep intimacy vibrant through different seasons of marriage?

DISCUSSION 1. COMMUNICATION BREAKDOWNS

Andre and Alisha

When Andre and Alisha first started trying to talk about intimacy, the conversations often felt awkward and frustrating. Alisha would share that she wanted to feel more connected, and Andre would hear this as a list of things he was doing wrong. He'd get tense, the conversation would stall, and they'd both walk away feeling misunderstood. After a while, Andre started keeping his thoughts to himself, hoping to avoid another uncomfortable exchange. Alisha noticed the distance and felt unsure how to bridge it, and their physical connection began to feel less natural.

One evening after a date, sitting in the car before heading home, Alisha tried something different. Instead of leading with what felt missing, she shared something that already mattered to her. "I really love when you hold my hand," she said. "It helps me feel close to you." Andre's tension eased. The conversation didn't magically fix everything, but it shifted the tone. They began to realize that how they talked about intimacy mattered just as much as what they were talking about, and that small changes in approach could make these conversations feel safer for both of them.

Mind

Intimacy is built on understanding, and understanding can't happen without healthy communication, but when conversations about sex feel awkward, tense, or unsafe, many couples default to avoiding the topic altogether. This avoidance creates mental distance, leaving one or both partners feeling unheard or misunderstood. Research shows that couples who regularly talk about their sexual relationship, both their needs and boundaries, report higher relationship satisfaction and more frequent intimacy.[1] This kind of open dialogue starts in the mind, with a willingness to be curious rather than critical, and to approach your spouse as a teammate instead of an adversary.

Body

When communication breaks down, your body often follows. Stress from unresolved tension activates the body's stress response, tightening muscles, increasing heart rate, and making it harder to physically relax with your spouse.[2] On the other hand, research shows that positive, supportive touch during conversations can help regulate stress and improve cooperation between partners.[3] A gentle hand squeeze or sitting close while talking sends a clear message: I'm with you, even if this is hard to talk about.

Soul

Proverbs 18:21 reminds us that "the tongue has the power of life and death." Words can build trust, or they can tear it down. In God's design, communication in marriage is not just about exchanging information. It's about reflecting His character in the way we speak and listen. James 1:19 calls us to be "quick to listen, slow to speak, and slow to become angry." When you choose to slow down, listen fully, and respond with grace, you are not just improving your intimacy, you are embodying the love of Christ to your spouse.

Questions

1. How comfortable am I currently talking about intimacy with my spouse?

____
____
____
____

2. When was the last time I felt truly heard in a conversation about my needs?

____
____
____
____

3. What is one small change I could make to help my spouse feel more understood?

____
____
____
____

PRACTICAL TIP

Set aside ten minutes this week for a no-logistics check-in: no talk about schedules, chores, or kids. Use that time to ask one curiosity question about your spouse's inner world or how to best communicate with him or her.

Prayer Prompt

Lord, help us speak life into our marriage. Give us courage to be honest; grace to listen well; and humility to seek understanding over being right.

DISCUSSION 2. DESIRE DIFFERENCES

Sofia and Lucas

Lucas loved pursuing his wife, Sofia, but lately, every time he reached for her, Sofia seemed to pull away. It wasn't that she didn't love him—she did—but between long workdays, the demands of caring for their toddler, and the changes in her body since childbirth, her desire just wasn't there. Each time she said, "Not tonight," Lucas felt more rejected, until eventually he stopped trying. He told himself it was easier to give up than to feel unwanted again.

One evening, Sofia noticed the quiet distance between them and finally asked: "Why don't you initiate anymore?" Lucas hesitated, then admitted: "Because every 'no' makes me feel like you don't want me." Tears filled her eyes. She hadn't realized how her "not now" was being heard as "not ever." They sat in silence for a moment, then Sofia whispered, "I don't want to push you away. I just don't know how to want it the way you do."

That conversation became a turning point. Together, without judgement, they began to explore what might be affecting Sofia's desire, including stress, fatigue, and even hormonal changes after pregnancy. With encouragement from Lucas, she booked an appointment with her doctor, who suggested checking hormone levels and exploring pelvic health therapy for lingering discomfort. At the same time that Sofia started pelvic health therapy and topical testosterone for low testosterone, she and Lucas made small, intentional choices to reconnect, such as cuddling without expectations, taking evening walks, and praying together before bed. Over time, the pressure began to lift, and intimacy started to feel like something they could discover together again, instead of something at which they were failing.

Mind

Desire starts in your brain, and not everyone's brain works in the same fashion. For some, desire is spontaneous, appearing almost out of nowhere like a flame from a spark in dry kindling. For others, desire is responsive and needs warmth, emotional connection, or specific cues before it catches fire. Neuroscience has shown these are simply two different patterns in the brain's arousal system, both designed by God.[4] One isn't better than the other; they just follow different starting points. In marriage, learning how your spouse's mind works and adjusting your expectations are challenges and opportunities and can help you see that variations in desire are not a reflection on you but simply reflect the way each person is wired.

One of the most common intimacy challenges in marriage is when one spouse wants sex more often than the other. This mismatch doesn't automatically mean something is wrong. Variation in human desire is normal. What makes the difference is how couples interpret and respond to this difference. When mismatched desire is met with criticism, pressure, or withdrawal, both partners can feel rejected or inadequate, but when it's approached with curiosity and grace, it becomes an opportunity to grow in empathy and creativity. Research shows that understanding your own and your spouse's desire style (whether spontaneous or responsive) helps reduce conflict and increases satisfaction for both partners.[5]

When repeated rejections pile up, it's easy for the initiating partner to quietly stop asking, not out of spite, but out of self-protection. The result is often a slow erosion of connection in which one feels unwanted and the other feels pressured. If you're the one saying no more often, it's worth exploring why you are saying no—not to blame yourself but to uncover what your body, mind, or spirit might be signaling. Low desire can stem from many causes: hormonal shifts (including menopause or postpartum changes), chronic stress, depression, certain medications, pelvic floor dysfunction, or unresolved relational tension. A medical provider can check hormone levels (such as testosterone, estrogen, and thyroid), review medications that may blunt desire, and refer to a pelvic health occupational or physical therapist for pain, tension, or mobility concerns. Sex counseling can also be helpful with desire concerns.

If you're the one who's stopped initiating, share openly that it's not about giving up but about protecting your heart—or whatever it is that you may be feeling. Then invite a conversation about how to find new ways to pursue intimacy without pressure. Remember, desire isn't "on" or "off"; it must be nurtured through emotional safety, playful connection, physical touch without an agenda, and addressing any underlying medical or relational barriers together.

Body

Your body's readiness for intimacy is influenced by stress, fatigue, and even the small signals you send each other throughout the day. For many with responsive desire, the body "switches on" after feeling seen, safe, and emotionally pursued. Research shows that consistent, non-demand touch (like holding hands, hugging, or sitting close) releases oxytocin, lowers cortisol, and makes the body more receptive to sexual connection.[6] Think of these small acts not as side notes but as the physical kindling that allows desire to grow.

Soul

Scripture invites us into a love that adapts and seeks the other's good. Philippians 2:3 calls us to "value others above yourselves," which includes learning your spouse's unique desire rhythm. God did not design marriage for perfect alignment. He designed it for love that leans in with humility and joy. Meeting your spouse's needs, whether that's creating emotional warmth first or responding to his or her spark, becomes an act of worship when done with a willing and submissive heart. This submission isn't one sided; it must be mutual.

Yes, mutual submission is biblical. Ephesians 5:21 reminds us to submit to one another out of reverence for Christ. In the realm of desire, this means that both husband and wife choose daily to honor each other, listen with patience, and offer grace when their rhythms do not match. In this shared posture, desire becomes less about performance and more about partnership.

Questions

1. Which type of desire (spontaneous or responsive) do I tend to experience most often?

____

____

____

____

2. What is one way my spouse could "light the kindling" for my desire this week?

____

____

____

____

3. When do I feel most emotionally open to intimacy, and what's happening in my body at that time (At ease? Excited? Relaxed? Increased blood flow to happy places?)?

____

____

____

____

PRACTICAL TIP

Identify one small, physical way to connect each day this week—without any expectation that it will lead to sex. Let the act be purely about connection. It could be an extended hug before leaving for work, snuggling on the couch for a set period of time, or holding hands after dinner. Decide together what it looks like and stick with it!

Prayer Prompt

Lord, thank You for designing us uniquely. Teach us to value each other's differences and pursue intimacy with kindness, patience, and joy.

DISCUSSION 3. BODY IMAGE AND SHAME

Carlos and Maria

After her second child was born, Maria often found herself standing in front of the mirror, tugging at her shirt and sighing. She loved her husband, Carlos, but she couldn't shake the thought: He must notice how much my body has changed. Whenever Carlos reached for her, she tensed. She wanted closeness, but her mind was already racing with self-criticism.

One evening, Carlos leaned in for a kiss, and she pulled back with a half-joke: "You don't want to see me right now." His confused face said it all: He wasn't seeing what she saw when she looked in the mirror. For him, her body wasn't something to be scrutinized but cherished. Unfortunately, Maria's inner dialogue had become so loud that it drowned out his affection.

Finally, after weeks of growing distance, Maria opened up to a close friend at church, who reminded her, "Your body is a temple, and it carried your babies. Can you thank God for that instead of fighting it?" That night, Maria tried something different. Before bed, instead of focusing on what she disliked, she prayed Psalm 139:14 over herself, thanking God for what her body could do: rock her children to sleep, hug her husband tight, and carry her through busy days. As she prayed, her breathing eased, her muscles softened, and intimacy began to feel possible again. Carlos recognized that Maria's shift in perspective helped her finally be present with him, unguarded and free.

Mind

How you think about your body directly shapes how you experience intimacy. If your inner dialogue is full of criticism—I've gained weight, I don't look like I used to, my spouse must notice every flaw—your brain stays in a guarded, self-monitoring mode instead of allowing you to relax and connect. This self-flagellation is often the result of years of cultural pressure, personal experiences, or even misunderstandings from early faith teaching that painted the body as shameful. Research has shown that practicing gratitude for your body, and focusing on what your body enables you to do rather than how it looks, can interrupt this mental loop, reducing self-objectification and increasing sexual satisfaction.[7]

Body

Shame isn't just in your head, it shows up physically. It can create muscle tension, shallow breathing, and lower arousal, sometimes even contributing to pain during intimacy. Your nervous system interprets self-criticism as a threat and responds by guarding rather than opening. Mindfulness-based body awareness, which involves slowing your breathing, noticing sensation without judgment, and focusing on physical connection, has been shown to reduce sexual distress and improve sexual function.[8] By gently retraining your body to relax in your spouse's presence, you can create the physical safety and openness needed for pleasure to flourish.

Soul

Psalm 139:14 reminds us: "I praise You because I am fearfully and wonderfully made." This is not just poetry; it is a theological truth about the value of your body as God's creation! We twist our perception of ourselves so that we hide, cover, and disconnect from the joy God intended. Practicing gratitude is more than a mental health tool; it's an act of worship and reclaiming. Every time you thank Him for your body, whether for the way your hands hold your spouse's, your legs carry you through the day, or your lungs draw breath, you resist shame and embrace God's truth.

Questions

1. How do I usually talk to myself about my body, and how does that affect my openness to intimacy?

2. What is one physical attribute or ability I can genuinely thank God for today?

3. How might shifting my focus from "how I look" to "what my body allows me to experience" change my intimacy?

PRACTICAL TIP

Each day this week, write down one thing that you're grateful your body can do. Keep the focus on function, connection, or experience over appearance.

Prayer Prompt

Lord, help me to see my body the way You do—good, purposeful, and worthy of love. Teach me to live in agreement with Your truth and to bring that freedom into my marriage.

DISCUSSION 4. STRESS, FATIGUE, AND MENTAL LOAD

Priya and Arjun

Arjun sat at the kitchen table long after his wife had gone to bed, laptop open, bills spread out, and tomorrow's work presentation running through his head. He wasn't avoiding her; he just felt empty. Every time Priya reached out, he pulled away—he loved her, but his mind was too full.

Over the past few months, Priya noticed the change. She thought maybe he wasn't attracted to her anymore. What she couldn't see was the invisible weight Arjun was carrying: late nights at work, worry over their oldest child struggling in school, and the endless mental to-do list that never seemed to shut off. By the time he crawled into bed, his body felt drained, and his mind was buzzing. Intimacy wasn't on the radar; survival was.

One Saturday, Priya suggested they go for a short hike instead of plowing through more chores. Arjun reluctantly agreed. Halfway through the walk, his shoulders began to unclench. He laughed for the first time in days, and by the end, he admitted, "I didn't realize how much I've been carrying." That evening, when they curled up together, the closeness came more easily. The stress did not disappear, but connection was still possible when Priya and Arjun made space to rest together instead of pushing harder.

Mind

Your brain is your biggest sex organ, and it's also the first to check out when it's overloaded. Chronic stress floods the body with cortisol, which suppresses sexual desire and disrupts arousal pathways in the brain.[9] The mental load many couples carry, such as tracking chores, kids' schedules, bills, and family needs, can quietly crowd out mental space for intimacy. This is especially true if one spouse carries more of the invisible planning and emotional management work, leading to resentment or emotional disconnection.[10] Understanding that stress and mental load aren't just mood killers but actual neurochemical factors helps couples approach this problem with teamwork instead of blame.

Body

Fatigue is more than being tired; it shifts your body into a conservation mode, prioritizing survival over connection. Research shows that even moderate chronic sleep loss changes levels of cortisol, insulin, and appetite-regulation hormones like ghrelin and leptin.[11] These shifts make it harder for the body to feel responsive or present in intimacy. Simple choices, like short walks, better sleep habits, or more affectionate touch when you're both more rested, can help restore your body's readiness for connection.

Soul

God designed intimacy to be a place of refreshment, not another source of pressure. In Matthew 11:28–30, Jesus invites the weary to come to Him for rest, an invitation that applies to every area of life, including marriage. When both spouses are stretched thin, pursuing intimacy requires a shift from performing to resting together. This might mean lowering expectations in some seasons, focusing on connection instead of frequency, and inviting God into the daily burdens that keep you from each other. Your soul and your intimacy can't thrive under constant strain.

Questions

1. What types of stress or responsibilities most often pull my focus away from intimacy?

2. How do we each experience and carry the mental load in our marriage?

____

____

____

____

3. What's one area where I could intentionally share or reduce a burden this week?

____

____

____

____

PRACTICAL TIP

Pick one evening this week to intentionally set aside the to-do list—no heavy conversations, no multi-tasking, just a shared activity you both find relaxing.

Prayer Prompt

Lord, teach us to lay down what we can't carry alone. Help us make space in our minds, bodies, and hearts for each other. Let our intimacy be a place of rest, joy, and renewal.

DISCUSSION 5. PERFORMANCE PRESSURE

Malik and Nia

Malik and Nia had been married for twelve years, but lately intimacy had started to feel more like a test than a joy. Every time they tried to be close, Malik found himself overthinking, wondering if he was doing everything right, if Nia was satisfied, if he was measuring up. The more he tried to control the moment, the more his body resisted. Frustration grew, and he often withdrew in silence afterward. Nia, meanwhile, worried she wasn't attractive to Malik anymore. What was meant to bring them together instead slowly built walls of misunderstanding.

Malik decided to try something different. Instead of trying again and ending in tension, they lit a candle and sat on the couch just to talk. Malik finally admitted, "I feel like every time we're together, I'm under a microscope. I want so badly to please you that I can't relax, and then it all falls apart. I've been under so much pressure to perform at work, I can't be under that same pressure at home, too." Nia's eyes filled with tears. "I never wanted you to feel that way," she said. "I don't need you to prove anything. I just want to feel close to you."

That conversation became a turning point. Together, they agreed to:

- **Remove the goal.** They practiced being affectionate without needing it to culminate in sex. Just touching, kissing, and enjoying time without pressure would be sufficient.
- **Try sensate focus.** Over a few weeks, they explored intentional nonsexual touch, from back massages to simply holding hands, retraining their bodies to relax into presence instead of bracing for pressure. (Sensate focus is described in detail in Part 3 of this guide.)
- **Slow down.** Malik began breathing more deeply, focusing on Nia's eyes, and noticing small sensations instead of trying to perform.
- **Reframe spiritually.** Before intimacy, they prayed together, asking God to remind them that sex was about connection, not accomplishment.

After several weeks, the heaviness began to lift. Malik and Nia laughed more. They touched more playfully. Not every moment was perfect, but they didn't need it to be. Malik said later, "Once I stopped trying to ace a test, I started enjoying being with my wife again."

Ana and Daniel

Ana and Daniel had been married for nearly a decade, but Ana often felt a weight hanging over their intimacy. From the start of their marriage, she believed she had to perform for Daniel and make sure she reached orgasm every time. If she didn't, she worried Daniel would feel inadequate, or worse, think something was wrong with her.

This pressure only grew stronger because of the messages Ana had absorbed from her upbringing. In her church youth group, sex had been framed as both a reward and a duty. It was something a good wife gave freely to her husband.

Since marrying Daniel, Ana didn't feel she had the space to talk about her own desires, rhythms, or needs. As a result, when she struggled to orgasm, Ana often felt broken, ashamed, and anxious.

The more she worried, the harder sex became. Instead of being present with Daniel, she found herself stuck in her own head, silently critiquing her body, replaying old messages about what sex was supposed to look like, and wondering why she couldn't relax. The cycle of pressure and disappointment left her dreading intimacy; she loved Daniel, but the bedroom had become a place of fear.

One evening, through tears, Ana finally told Daniel the burden she'd been carrying. To her surprise, he didn't respond with frustration or judgment. Instead, he reassured her: "I don't need you to perform for me. I just want you, the real you, not a perfect version." That conversation began to shift things. They slowed down, took the pressure off orgasm as the goal, and started focusing on connection, safety, and playfulness.

For Ana, one verse became a lifeline: "There is no fear in love, but perfect love drives out fear" (1 John 4:18). Slowly, she began to see intimacy as a safe space where fear didn't get the final word, not a test she had to pass. With Daniel's patience and God's grace, Ana learned that she wasn't broken at all! She was deeply loved, just as she was.

Mind

When intimacy becomes more about performance than connection, your mind can hijack the experience. The pressure to perform perfectly, whether sexually, emotionally, or spiritually, can create anxiety that blocks desire altogether. Research highlights that sexual performance anxiety significantly affects both partners, triggering cognitive distractions, physiological stress, and reduced satisfaction.[12] Understanding that these anxious thoughts are common, and not a moral failure, helps change your mindset from "should" and "must" to "safe space and closeness."

When intimacy feels like a test you have to pass, it shifts from connection to performance. Performance pressure can trigger the body's stress response, narrowing focus, increasing self-monitoring, and making it harder to relax into the moment.[13] This pressure often grows from internalized expectations, ideas about what intimacy should look like, frequency quotas, or the belief that your worth as a spouse hinges on meeting all these things. Sexual intimacy thrives when the mind is free from constant self-evaluation, allowing space for curiosity, play, and mutual enjoyment.

Body

Performance pressure isn't just mental; it shows up physiologically. Nervousness during intimacy raises cortisol, which reduces arousal, especially in women, and men aren't immune to this response either.[14] When your body's stress response is activated, desire and relaxation can vanish. Slowing down, leaning in, and using techniques like sensate focus, which refocuses connection beyond goals, can ease performance anxiety and create safe bodily space for intimacy.

The body doesn't distinguish between good pressure and bad pressure—it just knows when you're tense. For some men, this can result in difficulty maintaining erections; for some women, it can trigger pelvic floor tightening or reduced lubrication. Over time, repeated pressure-filled experiences can condition the body to anticipate failure, making arousal even harder to access.[15] Support from a pelvic health occupational or physical therapist can help retrain physical patterns, while strategies like slower pacing, breathwork, or focusing on pleasurable sensations (rather than end goals) can release unnecessary strain.

Soul

Scripture frames intimacy as sacred expression, not a show. In 1 Corinthians 7:3–5, marital intimacy is described as mutual care, not obligation or perfection. Intimacy is meant to be generous, not transactional. Letting go of performance pressure creates space to rest in identity and connection, not in accomplishment. When your soul embraces that intimacy is about giving and receiving love, not proving something, you invite grace and genuine closeness into your marriage.

Questions

1. In what moments do I feel most "on the clock" during intimacy?

____

____

____

____

2. How does the thought of "getting it right" affect my body's response?

____

____

____

____

3. What steps can we take together to reduce expectations and prioritize simply being together?

____

____

____

____

PRACTICAL TIP

Try a simplified sensate focus session this week. Set aside fifteen minutes to be near each other, holding hands, hugging, or caressing, without any goal or expectation for sex. Let the touch itself be the invitation.

Prayer Prompt

Lord, help us relinquish the pressure to perform. Teach us to receive each other as cherished gifts, trusting that intimacy grows best in the soil of grace, not performance.

DISCUSSION 6. PHYSICAL PAIN AND DYSFUNCTION

Ben and Mei

Mei had entered menopause five years earlier, and while hot flashes eventually subsided, intimacy became a different kind of challenge. Her vaginal tissue felt thinner and more fragile now, and what used to bring pleasure often left her feeling raw and uncomfortable. Ben, her husband of thirty-two years, still longed to be physically close every two or three days. For him, intimacy was a way of feeling connected and reassured. For Mei, that pace left her feeling sore, drained, and anxious about the next time.

At first, she kept quiet, bracing herself through the discomfort because she didn't want Ben to feel rejected. Over time, her body grew tense at even the thought of sex. She found herself pulling away from affectionate touches because she feared where they might lead. Ben, sensing the distance, grew frustrated and worried. His internal dialogue was brewing: I feel like you don't want me anymore.

One night, after another tearful conversation, Mei finally put words to what she was experiencing: "It's not that I don't want you. It's that my body feels sore for days after, and I can't keep up at this pace." For the first time, Ben heard pain, not rejection. He realized his longing for closeness had unintentionally pushed Mei into a cycle of discomfort and withdrawal.

Together, they sought help. Mei's gynecologist explained genitourinary syndrome of menopause (GSM), describing how lowered estrogen can thin and dry the vaginal tissue. She prescribed a low-dose vaginal estrogen cream and recommended lubricants designed for sensitive skin. The gynecologist also encouraged them to consider other ways of connecting physically that didn't always have to involve intercourse.

Ben agreed that they should stretch out the time between sexual encounters, and they began building intimacy through slower, non-penetrative touch, shared showers, and simply lying close together. Over time, Mei's comfort improved with treatment, and she felt safer knowing Ben valued her well-being over a rigid frequency.

Looking back, Mei reflected, "When I stopped hiding my pain, it freed us. Intimacy stopped being a chore and started feeling tender again." Ben admitted, "I thought what I needed was more sex, but what I really needed was to know we hadn't lost each other."

Mind

When intimacy hurts, it's not "all in your head," but your mind does shape how your body experiences pain. Anticipating discomfort can create a cycle of anxiety, muscle tension, and reduced desire, which actually heightens pain perception.[16] This can be especially true for women navigating menopause or postpartum recovery, where hormonal changes may already affect comfort. For some couples, fear of pain leads to avoiding intimacy altogether, unintentionally widening emotional distance. Recognizing that pain is a signal, not a sentence, can help you shift from self-blame to problem-solving together.

YOU ARE NOT A PIECE OF CHEWED-UP GUM

If you grew up in church youth groups in the 1990s or early 2000s, you may remember an object lesson that went something like this: A piece of gum was passed around the room. Each time someone "chewed" it, the gum became less appealing. The message was clear and graphic. Every sexual thought, touch, or experience supposedly made you less desirable. By the end, no one would want what had already been "used."

This kind of teaching is often referred to as being part of *purity culture*, a framework that defined sexual faithfulness primarily through fear, avoidance, and external behavior rather than formation, wisdom, or mutuality.

We want to be clear: Purity culture's fear-mongering, shame-inducing messages are not okay, and those messages do **not** reflect God's heart. Comparing people, especially girls or women, to pieces of chewed-up gum reduces people made in God's image to objects to be used up or discarded, rather than whole persons meant to be known, respected, and safe in relationships. Purity culture aimed to scare teenagers into purity. Instead, it planted shame deep in many people's bodies.

For some, purity culture led to rushing into marriage before being emotionally ready. They believed sex would instantaneously become good on the wedding night once they had the "all clear." For others, the sudden switch from "sex equals bad" to "sex equals holy" felt jarring and confusing, leaving their nervous systems unsure how to respond. Some people didn't wait until marriage and felt permanently "ruined," questioning their worth, their faith, or both. For many women, those harmful messages didn't just stay in their minds. The messages of shame and distrust of one's own body became literally embodied as pain with penetration, vaginismus, pelvic floor tension, inability to orgasm, or a body that simply would not relax, even when they were with someone they deeply loved.

The good news? None of that means you are broken.

Those responses of pain and discomfort are often your body doing exactly what it learned to do: protect you from something you were taught to fear. Shame may have been preached as holiness, but God does not compare you to a piece of chewed-up gum. God's design for intimacy is about being fully known and trusted, where connection grows through mutual care and shared delight.

If you see yourself in any of these examples, know this: Healing is possible. Your body can learn safety. Pleasure can become a pathway to feeling at home in your own body. Intimacy can be rebuilt slowly with care, consent, and compassion. You are not less because of your past. You are not used. You are whole, beloved, and worthy of intimacy that honors both your body and your soul.

Body

Pain during intimacy can have many causes: pelvic floor muscle dysfunction, hormonal shifts in menopause, postpartum healing and hormones, chronic illness, arthritis, autoimmune disorders, medication side effects, or more. For women, conditions like vulvodynia, vaginismus, and endometriosis may contribute. For men, erectile dysfunction or pelvic pain disorders can create similar challenges. Evidence shows that working with a pelvic health occupational or physical therapist can significantly reduce pain, improve pelvic floor function, and restore comfort, in addition to getting help from a medical doctor, physician assistant, nurse practitioner, or certified nurse midwife.[17] These providers address muscle tension, scar tissue mobility, hormonal considerations, and body awareness, helping you move toward pain-free connection.

Soul

Physical challenges in intimacy can leave you feeling broken or less than, but Scripture tells a different story. Job testifies, "You clothed me with skin and flesh and knit me together with bones and sinews" (Job 10:11), reminding you that your body was formed with care and intention. Even when your body feels unfamiliar or unreliable, God has not forgotten how He made you. There is also a beautiful promise found in Isaiah: "Even to your old age and gray hairs I am He, I am He who will sustain you. I have made you and I will carry you; I will sustain you and I will rescue you" (Isaiah 46:4). Seasons of physical difficulty can become opportunities to grow in empathy, patience, and creativity in your marriage. Intimacy is not limited to one expression. It's about unity, tenderness, and mutual joy, even as you pursue healing.

GENITOURINARY SYNDROME OF MENOPAUSE (AND RELATED SEASONS)

During menopause, postpartum recovery, and lactation, many women experience lower estrogen levels. This shift affects desire as well as the health of genitourinary tissues. Collectively, this cluster of changes is known as *genitourinary syndrome of menopause,* or GSM.

- **Desire:** Hormonal shifts can lower libido and decrease genital blood flow, making arousal more difficult.

- **Tissue health:** Vaginal tissues may become thinner, less elastic, and less lubricated. This can make penetration uncomfortable or even painful.

- **Comfort and risk:** Dryness and fragile tissue increase the risk of micro-tears, bleeding, or recurrent urinary tract infections.

- **When to seek help:** Simple interventions like vaginal moisturizers, lubricants, low-dose vaginal estrogen, or other hormone or non-hormone therapies can dramatically improve comfort and sexual well-being. These should always be discussed with a qualified medical provider.

Pain with sex is not just part of getting older. Solutions exist! Seeking care from a pelvic health occupational or physical therapist can restore both comfort and confidence in intimacy.

Questions

1. How does the possibility or presence of pain affect my emotional readiness for intimacy?

____

____

____

____

2. What steps could we take together to better understand and address any physical challenges?

____

____

____

____

3. How can we stay connected while one or both of us is healing?

____

____

____

____

PRACTICAL TIP

Create a shared "comfort menu" of physical touches, activities, and settings you both enjoy when intimacy is tender or limited. Include options for different moods, such as cuddling with a blanket, slow dancing in the kitchen, a warm bath together, or gentle massage. Keep it handy so you can choose from it during connection times without pressure.

Prayer Prompt

Lord, thank You for crafting our bodies with care. Give us the courage to seek help, the patience to heal, and the creativity to connect in ways that nurture joy and closeness.

DISCUSSION 7. RESENTMENT AND UNRESOLVED CONFLICT

Ruth and Calvin

Calvin had been looking forward to the weekend for weeks. He had booked a cozy cabin two hours away, arranged childcare for the kids, and even mapped out a few hikes and dinner spots. His hope was simple: reconnect with Ruth and rekindle a spark that had been dulled by months of busyness.

When they finally arrived at the cabin, Ruth's phone kept buzzing with work emails, texts from friends, and updates about the kids. It seemed as if her attention was anywhere but with him. Calvin tried to brush it off at first, telling himself, She's just overwhelmed; give her time.

By the third time she checked her notifications during what was supposed to be a quiet, romantic dinner, Calvin's chest tightened. Instead of leaning in, he withdrew. His mind began replaying all the ways he had felt pushed to the side in recent months. He had poured energy into planning something special, but her distracted glances at the glowing screen felt like rejection. That night, though Ruth reached for him in bed, Calvin hesitated. Resentment whispered, "Why should I give more when she doesn't value me?"

For the rest of the weekend, Calvin carried that unspoken weight. Ruth noticed his distance but misinterpreted it as lack of desire. The silence between them grew louder than any words they exchanged.

Finally, on the drive home, Calvin broke and said, "I wanted this weekend to be about us, but it felt like your phone was more important." Ruth's eyes welled up. She hadn't realized how deeply her distraction had affected him. She replied, "I thought I was keeping things under control so I could relax with you. I didn't see how it looked from your side."

That conversation marked the beginning of a shift. Ruth agreed to set clearer boundaries with her phone, especially during time meant for connection. She silenced her work notifications after 6:00 p.m., kept her phone out of reach during meals, and she left her phone out of the bedroom at night by switching to a separate alarm clock. Calvin learned to name his hurt before it hardened into distance. They didn't fix everything in one car ride, but by addressing the resentment, they took a step toward rebuilding both trust and intimacy.

Mind

Lingering resentment resembles mental clutter: You might not notice it every moment, but it shapes how you respond, interpret, and connect. Neuroscience shows that when we hold onto negative emotions toward our spouse, our brain's stress response stays activated, making empathy and desire harder to access.[18] Even small, unresolved issues can build a mental distance that turns warmth into defensiveness.

Recognizing resentment doesn't mean dwelling on it. Instead, focus on identifying the resentment's root issue so you can work together to resolve the problem.

Body

Emotional disconnection doesn't just live in your mind; it shows up in your body. Chronic unresolved tension can elevate cortisol, increase muscle tightness, and even reduce arousal responses.[19] This can make intimacy feel forced or undesirable, reinforcing the cycle of distance. Over time, your body learns to associate your spouse's presence with vigilance rather than relaxation. Restoring the emotional bond often brings physical relief, lower stress, softer touch, and greater openness to pleasure.

Soul

Scripture doesn't shy away from the danger of unresolved conflict. Ephesians 4:26–27 urges us not to let the sun go down while we're still angry, "and do not give the devil a foothold." Resentment creates fertile ground for division in marriage, but reconciliation brings life. God calls us to forgive as we have been forgiven (Colossians 3:13), not to excuse harm, but to release the burden that blocks intimacy. Healing may take time, but every step toward grace reclaims unity that reflects Christ's love.

Questions

1. What unresolved frustrations might still be affecting how we connect physically or emotionally?

____

____

____

____

2. How do we each tend to handle conflict? Is it through avoidance, escalation, or do we work toward reconnection?

____

____

____

____

3. What would rebuilding trust and warmth look like for us right now?

____

____

____

____

PRACTICAL TIP

Schedule a fifteen- to twenty-minute reset time once a week to air small frustrations before they pile up. Use a simple format: (1) share something you appreciated this week, (2) share one thing that hurt or frustrated you, and (3) suggest one change that would help you feel more connected. End with prayer or a hug to close the loop.

Prayer Prompt

Lord, help us to release resentment and seek reconciliation. Give us humble hearts, listening ears, and the courage to restore what's been strained so our marriage reflects Your grace.

DISCUSSION 8. HEALING FROM PAST SEXUAL WOUNDS

Adam and Layla

Adam grew up hearing two very different messages about sex. From society, he absorbed the idea that a "real man" should always want sex and that a satisfying marriage meant frequent, adventurous intimacy. From church, he often heard purity culture messages that sex was bad or dangerous before marriage, but afterward, it would be effortless, frequent, and deeply fulfilling if you just "did things God's way."

By the time Adam married Layla, those messages had fused into one expectation: that intimacy would come naturally, frequently, and almost on demand. At first, he was excited to explore sex with his new wife, but when Layla sometimes hesitated or wasn't immediately responsive, he felt confused and even rejected. In his mind, intimacy had been promised as a reward for waiting, so why didn't it look like the fantasy he had carried for years?

This gap between expectation and reality slowly took a toll. Adam began to keep a quiet scorecard in his head: how many days it had been, how often Layla said yes, and how long it took her to seem interested or physically responsive once intimacy was initiated. He didn't notice it at first, but his focus on frequency over connection created distance. Layla sensed the pressure and started feeling like intimacy was a chore, not a delight. Adam, in turn, felt more frustrated and began withdrawing emotionally.

One evening, after an argument sparked by his disappointment when Layla wasn't in the mood, she asked, "Adam, do you really want me, or do you just want sex?" The words stung, but they cut through the fog. Adam realized his expectations had been shaped more by culture and church slogans than by love, patience, or mutual care.

With time, counseling with a mental health care professional, and prayer, Adam began to unlearn those scripts. He and Layla started having honest conversations about what intimacy meant to both of them physically, emotionally, and spiritually. He learned to see intimacy as an overflow of connection, not a scoreboard to measure success. Passages like Ephesians 5:25, "Husbands, love your wives, just as Christ loved the Church and gave Himself up for her," taught him that love was not about demand but about sacrifice and service.

As Adam let go of rigid expectations, Layla felt safer and more desired as a whole person. Slowly, intimacy became less about performance and frequency, and more about joy, tenderness, and partnership. Adam realized that God wasn't interested in rewarding a transactional view of sex. He was interested in shaping a love that reflected Christ's heart.

Mind

Past sexual wounds, whether from trauma, betrayal, or harmful teaching, can rewire the brain's responses to intimacy. Trauma activates the amygdala (the brain's alarm system) making it more likely for a person to experience hypervigilance, intrusive thoughts, or emotional shutdown during closeness.[20] Shame-based sexual teaching can also form deep mental scripts that link intimacy with fear, guilt, or danger. These mental associations can create a cycle where sexual connection feels unsafe, even with a loving spouse. Healing begins with recognizing that these are learned patterns that, with God's help, can be gently replaced through new experiences of safety, respect, and love.

Body

Sexual trauma and long-term shame don't just live in the mind, they leave imprints in the body. Survivors often have heightened sympathetic nervous system responses, pelvic floor overactivity, or changes in hormonal regulation that affect arousal and comfort.[21] For women, pelvic health occupational or physical therapy can address muscle tension, scar tissue, and hypersensitivity. This is especially important during life stages like postpartum recovery or menopause, when hormonal changes can increase discomfort.[22] For men, trauma can contribute to erectile dysfunction or difficulty with orgasm because of chronic stress responses. Gentle, graded exposure to nonsexual touch, paired with regulated breathing and grounding techniques, can help retrain the body to associate intimacy with safety and pleasure.

Soul

Past wounds distort God's good design for intimacy, but Scripture promises that "He heals the brokenhearted and binds up their wounds" (Psalm 147:3). Sexual connection was created by God to be a place of unity, delight, and mutual blessing within marriage (Song of Songs 4:9–10). The gospel reminds us that, in Christ, our past does not define our worth, our identity, or our ability to give and receive love. Healing is not about erasing the past; it's about letting the Holy Spirit rewrite the ending, redeeming what was stolen and restoring joy where there was once pain.

Questions

1. How have past experiences or teachings shaped the way I approach intimacy today?

____

____

____

____

2. What helps me feel emotionally and physically safe with my spouse?

____

____

____

____

3. How can we invite God into our healing process together as a couple?

____

____

____

____

PRACTICAL TIP

Pick one short moment this week to replace a triggering or shaming thought about your body or past with a truth from Scripture. First, notice the thought ("I'm damaged goods"). Then, use a concordance, Bible app, or simple web search like "Bible verses about [keyword]" to find a verse that speaks truth into that specific fear or lie. For example, for shame about your body, you might meditate on 1 Corinthians 6:19–20, which reminds us that our bodies are temples of the Holy Spirit and that we were "bought at a price." Pause, breathe deeply once, and repeat your chosen verse out loud. This quick swap gently retrains your brain, calms your body's stress response, and anchors your spirit in God's truth.

Prayer Prompt

Lord, You know the wounds we carry, and You promise to be close to the brokenhearted. Help us walk this healing journey together, replacing fear with trust and shame with Your truth. Restore what's been lost and help us see each other through Your eyes.

DISCUSSION 9. FAITH AND INTIMACY INTEGRATION

Esther and Chris

Esther and Chris had been married for over twenty years. Their love was steady, but intimacy often felt like a quiet duty, something they assumed was good and necessary, but not necessarily thrilling. Esther sometimes whispered to herself, "Maybe this is all God meant sex to be—simple and practical."

Then, during a Bible study on Song of Songs, they were stunned. For the first time, they noticed how openly Scripture described marital passion not as ordinary, but as breathtaking. They read words like, "How delightful is your love, my sister, my bride! How much more pleasing is your love than wine" (Song of Songs 4:10). Chris blinked at the verse, then turned to Esther: "This doesn't sound like duty. This sounds—mind-blowing."

That realization reframed everything. They began to see intimacy as a sacred gift designed by God to be full of delight, creativity, and even playfulness, not a chore. Esther felt free to let go of old inhibitions rooted in the idea that pleasure was somehow selfish. Chris realized he didn't have to downplay desire; in fact, God celebrated it.

One night, instead of rushing through the familiar script, they slowed down, laughing, touching, and exploring in ways that they hadn't in years. For the first time in decades, Esther thought, God actually wants this to be amazing. The joy and closeness they felt that evening was unlike anything they'd expected at this stage of marriage.

They realized God's design for intimacy was never meant to be bland or just enough. He created it to be abundant, passionate, and life-giving—a physical echo of His extravagant love.

Mind

Sexual intimacy is more than just a physical act; it is a deeply integrated expression of emotional, relational, and spiritual connection. From a psychological perspective, meaning and purpose in intimacy strengthen relationship satisfaction, trust, and resilience. When couples see intimacy as a part of God's good design for their union, not just meeting a need, it shifts the focus from performance to connection. Studies have shown that when sexual experiences are imbued with emotional and spiritual meaning, couples report greater satisfaction and less relational stress.[23] Understanding that your physical connection can serve as a form of worship (an act of giving and receiving love as God intended) helps reframe intimacy as a shared mission rather than a mere event.

Body

Our bodies are designed for connection. Physically, sexual touch releases oxytocin and other bonding hormones that reinforce feelings of closeness and safety.

From a pelvic health perspective, cultivating an environment of meaning and emotional safety can reduce physical tension and improve arousal. This is particularly important during seasons of change (such as menopause) when hormonal shifts can affect desire and comfort. Integrating a holistic view of intimacy can help couples approach physical changes as opportunities to explore new ways of giving and receiving pleasure that honor both partners' bodies.

Soul

Scripture reveals God's delight in marital intimacy! It was never meant to be seen as something shameful or hidden, but as a reflection of His covenant love. In Song of Songs, we see passion, playfulness, and mutual delight celebrated. The act of coming together physically can be a reminder of the spiritual covenant you've entered into before God—a renewal of your "one flesh" union (Genesis 2:24). When you view intimacy as a spiritual practice, it becomes about reinforcing the God-given mission and purpose of your marriage, not just personal enjoyment. In this light, sex is not disconnected from faith but is a tangible way of living it out.

Questions

1. How does viewing intimacy as part of our shared spiritual mission change the way we approach it?

____

____

____

____

2. In what ways could we make our physical connection feel more purposeful and meaningful?

____

____

____

____

3. What biblical truths challenge or reshape the way we've been taught to think about marital intimacy?

____

____

____

____

MALE GENITAL AND HORMONAL CHANGES THAT AFFECT INTIMACY

Although men don't experience a menopause, they do experience age-related and health-related changes that can affect desire and function. These are sometimes called *androgen decline in aging males* (ADAM) or simply late-onset hypogonadism.

- **Desire:** Declining testosterone levels can reduce libido, energy, and confidence.

- **Erectile function:** Conditions like diabetes, cardiovascular disease, pelvic surgery, or certain medications (such as anti-hypertensives or SSRIs) can contribute to erectile dysfunction (ED).

- **Comfort and risk:** ED can create frustration, avoidance, or relational strain; medications or mechanical aids (such as vacuum devices) can help. Men with low testosterone or persistent ED should be evaluated, because these can also flag larger health concerns (such as cardiac, metabolic, or endocrine issues).

- **When to seek help:** Ask a provider about hormone testing, ED medications (such as PDE5 inhibitors), pelvic health occupational or physical therapy, or addressing underlying health conditions.

Needing help with arousal or erections is common and treatable. Early conversations with a provider can open doors to safe and effective support for both partners.

PRACTICAL TIP

This week, set aside one intentional moment (outside the bedroom) to talk with your spouse about what intimacy means to you beyond the physical. Share how you believe it strengthens your marriage's mission and reflects your faith. Then, choose one small physical expression of affection that carries that shared meaning such as a lingering hug, holding hands during prayer, or a slow dance in the kitchen.

Prayer Prompt

Lord, thank You for creating us to connect in body, mind, and spirit. Help us to see our intimacy as part of Your good design and our marriage's purpose. Give us wisdom to honor You through how we love one another in every way.

DISCUSSION 10. LONG-TERM SPARK

José and Renee

When José and Renee's youngest child moved out, their house suddenly felt quiet in a way that was both strange and freeing. For years, their energy had gone into raising children, juggling work, and keeping the family running smoothly. Now, for the first time in decades, it was just the two of them again.

At first, the silence felt awkward. Soon, they realized they had a gift: the chance to rediscover each other without distraction. They began by going on weekly date nights (and not just dinner!). They did things that made them laugh and play, such as cooking classes, hiking new trails, and even trying salsa dancing. Each experience reminded them of the curiosity and fun that had first drawn them together.

At home, they noticed the shift carried over into their intimacy. Without the constant demands of parenting, they could linger, experiment, and talk openly about what they enjoyed. Renee admitted she had felt overlooked during the busy years, and José confessed he had sometimes felt shut out. Naming those feelings brought healing, and the freedom of this new season allowed them to explore intimacy with fresh joy.

Spiritually, the words of Proverbs 5:18, "Rejoice in the wife of your youth," took on new meaning. José and Renee realized God hadn't designed intimacy to fade after the honeymoon or disappear in midlife. Instead, He intended it to deepen, mature, and even feel brand-new at times. For them, empty-nesting didn't signal the end of passion; it opened the door to a new honeymoon season.

Now, when their friends ask about this stage of marriage, José and Renee laugh and say, "It feels like we're dating again, except better, because we know each other's hearts so much more."

Mind

Over the course of marriage, life inevitably changes, careers shift, children grow up, health challenges arise, and seasons of stress or transition come and go. Novelty and emotional connection stimulate the brain's reward system, strengthening attraction and bonding.[24] Novelty doesn't have to mean something wild or exotic. It can simply mean new shared experiences, intentional curiosity about each other, and fresh ways of expressing love. By staying curious about your spouse in every season, you avoid letting familiarity turn into autopilot. God designed our relationships to grow and adapt, and our minds are capable of delighting in one another when we nurture that curiosity.

Body

Physical intimacy evolves over time. Hormonal shifts from aging, postpartum recovery, or menopause can influence arousal and comfort.[25] That's why it's important to adjust, not retreat. Couples thrive when they learn how to work with their changing bodies through gentle exploration, adapting positions, and building in extended warm-up time. Your body can remain a place of connection and joy when you give it grace for its season, rather than comparing it to a different chapter of your marriage.

Soul

From a spiritual perspective, intimacy is part of the lifelong covenant, not just the honeymoon phase. Scripture calls us to "rejoice in the wife of your youth" (Proverbs 5:18). You do not stay the same; your love matures and deepens. In every season, intimacy can be a living testimony of God's faithful love, grace that adapts, passion that renews, and joy that's rooted in something more lasting than feelings alone. Seeing your intimacy as part of your shared purpose in God's story transforms it from something you keep alive into something you continually grow.

Questions

1. What is new way we could connect this month that we've never tried before, physically, emotionally, or spiritually?

____

____

____

____

2. How have we seen our intimacy change for the better during our relationship?

____

____

____

____

3. What do we want our intimate connection to look and feel like in the next season of our marriage?

____

____

____

____

PRACTICAL TIP

Plan a micro-adventure together—a small, new experience that's just for the two of you. It could be as simple as trying a new coffee shop, going for a sunrise walk, or dancing in the living room to a song you've never heard before. Link this experience with some form of affectionate touch so that your brain and body associate novelty with connection.

Prayer Prompt

Lord, thank You for the gift of a love that changes and deepens with time. Help us to stay curious about each other, to embrace the seasons You bring, and to keep choosing connection—mind, body, and soul—no matter what life holds.

[1] E. Sandra Byers, "Relationship Satisfaction and Sexual Satisfaction: A Longitudinal Study of Individuals in Long-Term Relationships," *Journal of Sex Research* 42, no. 2 (2005): 113.

[2] Mattie Tops et al. "Rejection Sensitivity Relates to Hypocortisolism and Depressed Mood State in Young Women," *Psychoneuroendocrinology* 33, no. 4 (2008): 551.

[3] James A. Coan, Hillary S. Schaefer, and Richard J. Davidson, "Lending a Hand: Social Regulation of the Neural Response to Threat," *Psychological Science* 17, no. 12 (2006): 1038.

[4] Rosemary Basson, "A Model of Women's Sexual Arousal," *Journal of Sex & Marital Therapy* 28, no. 1 (2002): 9.

[5] Kristen P. Mark and Julie A. Lasslo, "Maintaining Sexual Desire in Long-Term Relationships: A Systematic Review and Conceptual Model," *Journal of Sex Research* 55, nos. 4–5 (2018): 14.

[6] Erin T. Fitzpatrick, et al. "Sexual Satisfaction Mediates Daily Associations between Body Satisfaction and Relationship Satisfaction in New Parent Couples," *Journal of Sex Research* 51, (2024): 101810.

[7] Kristin J. Homan and Tracy L. Tylka, "Appearance-Based Exercise Motivation Moderates the Relationship between Exercise Frequency and Positive Body Image," *Body Image* 11, no. 2 (2014): 107.

[8] Lori A. Brotto and Rosemary Basson, "Group Mindfulness-Based Therapy Significantly Improves Sexual Desire in Women," *Behavior Research and Therapy* 57 (2014): 52.

[9] Lisa Dawn Hamilton and Cindy M. Meston, "Chronic Stress and Sexual Function in Women," *Journal of Sexual Medicine* 10, no. 10 (2013): 2452.

[10] Allison Daminger, "The Cognitive Dimension of Household Labor," *American Sociological Review* 84, no. 4 (2019): 609.

[11] Rachel Leproult and Eve Van Cauter, "Role of Sleep and Sleep Loss in Hormonal Release and Metabolism," *Endocrine Development* 17 (2010): 17.

[12] Amanda Bockaj et al., "Under Pressure: Men's and Women's Sexual Performance Anxiety in the Sexual Interactions of Adult Couples," *Journal of Sex Research* 62, no. 8 (2025): 1450.

[13] *Ibid.*

[14] Lisa Dawn Hamilton, Alessandra H. Rellini, and Cindy M. Meston, "Cortisol, Sexual Arousal, and Affect in Response to Sexual Stimuli," *The Journal of Sexual Medicine* 5, no. 9 (2008): 2116.

[15] John Bancroft, *Human Sexuality and Its Problems,* 3rd ed. (Elsevier Health Sciences, 2008), 98.

[16] Stephanie Both, Walter Everaerd, and Ellen Laan, "Modulation of Spinal Reflexes by Aversive or Positive Sexual Stimuli," *Psychophysiology* 40, no. 2 (2003): 181.

[17] Małgorzata Starzec-Proserpio et al., "Effectiveness of Nonpharmacological Conservative Therapies for Chronic Pelvic Pain in Women: A Systematic Review and Meta-Analysis," *American Journal of Obstetrics and Gynecology* 232, no. 1 (2025): 42.

[18] Coan, "Lending a Hand," 1037.

[19] Hamilton et al., "Cortisol, Sexual Arousal," 2111.

[20] Bessel A. Van der Kolk, *The Body Keeps the Score: Brain, Mind, and Body in the Healing of Trauma* (Viking, 2014).

21 Alessandra H. Rellini, Lisa Dawn Hamilton, Yvon Delville, and Cindy M. Meston, "The Cortisol Response during Physiological Sexual Arousal in Women with and without a History of Childhood Sexual Abuse," *Journal of Traumatic Stress* 22, no. 6 (2009): 563.

22 Susan Wysocki, Sheryl A. Kingsberg, and Michael Krychman, "Management of Vulvar and Vaginal Atrophy: Implications from the REVIVE (Real Women's Views of Treatment Options for Menopausal Vaginal Changes) Survey," *Clinical Medicine Insights: Reproductive Health* 8 (2014): 24.

23 Woet L. Gianotten, Jenna C. Alley, and Lia M. Diamond, "The Health Benefits of Sexual Expression," *International Journal of Sexual Health* 33, no. 4 (2021): 10.

24 Bianca P. Acevedo and Arthur P. Aron, "Romantic Love, Pair-Bonding, and the Dopaminergic Reward System," in *Mechanisms of Social Connection: From Brain to Group,* ed. Mario Mikulincer and Phillip R. Shaver (American Psychological Association, 2014): 55.

25 Sheryl A. Kingsberg and Tamara Woodard, "Female Sexual Dysfunction: Focus on Low Desire," *Obstetrics and Gynecology* 125, no. 2 (2015): 477.

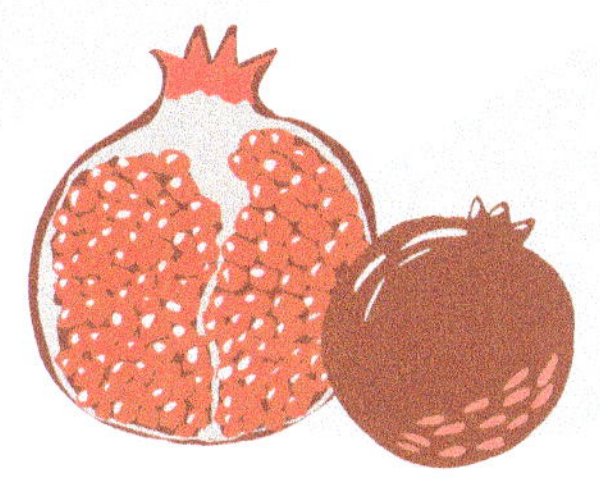

PART 3.
Putting Intimacy into Practice

HIGHLIGHTS

sensate focus • word play • hand skills • mouth skills • grounding
practice • pillows, props, and positions • sensory play • desire builders •
vibrators • mixing and matching practices • checking back in

Now what? Now that we are on the same page of what sexual function looks like, and we are feeling more connected, we've designed some practical activities for you to try out in the bedroom. There's no need to try them all at once—unless you've got the time or a beautiful hotel room that's setting the mood for play.

As we mentioned at the beginning of this guide, these practices are written for marriages that are safe, mutual, and life-giving. Intimacy flourishes when both husband and wife feel honored, heard, and free to say "no" (or "not yet") without fear of anger, manipulation, silence, or any kind of harm.

Sexual abuse and abuse happen in far too many marriages. You are worth safety, dignity, and care, and God hates the abuse of His daughters and sons. If any of the statements below feel true for you right now, please pause and reach out for help:

- You're afraid to say no or set a boundary.
- Touch (even non-sexual) often feels demanding or punishing.
- Past or present coercion, force, or any non-consensual act has occurred.
- You feel chronically small, guilty, or responsible for your spouse's emotions around sex.

You are not alone, and healing is possible. Start with a trusted pastor, licensed counselor, or call the National Domestic Violence Hotline (800-799-7233) or text "START" to 88788. When safety and mutual delight exist, these practices can be a source of beautiful connection. Until then, your well-being matters more than any exercise in this book. Please seek out any help you need.

PRACTICE 1. SENSATE FOCUS

Remember the first time you held each other's hands, and your palms got all sweaty because you were nervous, excited, and overwhelmed by new sensations? Yeah, we're going to flip that nervous energy around and turn touch into intimate knowing. **Sensate focus** (fancy therapist term) is basically a no-pressure, clothes-on (at first) way to rediscover every inch of each other as if it's the first time. For some of us, it still kind of is the first time to know our spouse in this way.

Your Step-by-Step Roadmap

1. Pick your night and protect it. Silence phones, lock the door, light a candle, or keep it dark. Set the environment to whatever helps you both exhale. Aim for thirty to forty-five minutes of uninterrupted time.
2. Decide who is the giver and who is the receiver first. Flip a coin, pray about it, or just take turns. The receiver keeps at least underwear on for the beginning, or even the whole time—whatever feels right for the receiver. Clothes come off only when both of you feel excited curiosity. Removing clothing should never be an obligation.
3. Set the ground rules together (say them out loud the first few times). Here are some examples:

- No breasts or genitals. This could be for a certain time period like the first five or ten minutes, or it could be for the entire session. Some couples find they get more in tune with their desire if breasts and genitals are off-limits the first time or two that they complete this practice. What matters is that you are talking about it.
- Feedback is welcome ("slower," "harder," "that tickles," "don't stop"), but no directing an entire performance.
- Receiver's job: Notice sensations and breathe. Giver's job: Touch as if you're exploring with sacred reverence.

4. The receiver gets comfy (lying down, sitting propped up, whatever feels safe). You can close your eyes if it helps you tune in better.

5. Giver begins the slow exploration. You can use dry hands first or jump straight to lotion or oil if your or the receiver's skin is dry. Here is a sample path for exploration. Stay as long as you both want on any spot:
   - Face, scalp, ears, neck
   - Shoulders, arms, hands (massage every finger)
   - Chest, sides of ribcage, belly
   - Back, lower back, buttocks (over clothes or bare)
   - Legs, inner thighs, feet

6. It's okay to stay here for as long as you need. For some, this is as far as it gets for a session. Some couples may be rediscovering intimacy together, and they camp out in the safe zones for weeks, and that's perfect. Staying on non-erogenous parts of the body can be especially helpful and common during postpartum recovery, menopause, illness, and so forth.

7. When (and only when) both of you feel ready to level up, you can move to more erogenous zones.
   - Include breasts or chest and buttocks
   - Then inner thighs and external genitals (no penetration required)
   - Then manual or oral stimulation to orgasm, if that's where the Spirit and your bodies lead you

8. Permission statements to say out loud if you need them:
   - "We can stop at any level tonight, and it's still a win."
   - "Orgasm is welcome if it happens, but it's never the goal."
   - "If one of us wants to keep clothes on longer, we both celebrate that boundary."

9. Receiver's job, every step of the way: Notice temperature, pressure, and texture. Breathe slowly. Let your body speak. What you are experiencing (goosebumps, sighs, giggles, tears, arousal) is all data—and none of that data is wrong. If your mind wanders to tomorrow's to-do list, gently come back to the fingertip that's loving you right now.

10. Switch roles. Repeat the exact same journey on your spouse. You'll be shocked how different the same touch feels when you're receiving.

11. Debrief: Three minutes of gold. Do not skip this step. Sit up, hold each other, and finish these statements:
    - "The touch that surprised me most was . . ."
    - "I felt most alive or connected when . . ."
    - "Next time I'd love more of _____ or less of _____." Keep the debrief grateful and short.

12. Progress at your own pace. No one is testing you here. There is no falling behind. Some couples go from fully clothed to mutual orgasm the first time they do this activity. Some take three months to go topless. Some decide oral or genital touch isn't their thing right now, and that's just as holy. This practice works at every single level because the real goal is naked and unashamed trust, not a checklist.

Sensate Focus When Bodies Are Tired, Healing, or Changing

Bodies and seasons change. After having a baby, during pain or healing, or through menopause, erectile dysfunction, low desire, stress, or deep exhaustion, intimacy can start to feel different than it once did. These changes can feel confusing or frustrating. There is hope; you are not broken. Sensate focus is especially helpful in these seasons because it meets tired, healing, or changing bodies with gentleness, flexibility, and care rather than pressure or performance.

- Stay in cozy pajamas, a nursing bra, or even socks if that feels safer.
- Use tools if hands feel too intense, such as a silk scarf dragged across skin, a soft makeup brush, a feather tickler, or the back of a cool spoon.
- The receiver can stay sitting propped with pillows or lying on his or her side. Do whatever protects your back, hips, or incision sites if you are feeling discomfort or need to adjust positions.

- You can focus on the scalp, hands, feet, neck, and outer arms or legs if the middle of the body doesn't feel ready for touch or exploration right now. These focus areas still light up the same pleasure pathways in the brain.
- If something hurts, leaks, or just won't relax, that's your body waving a little flag that says, "I need extra help." A pelvic health occupational or physical therapist can teach you gentle ways to calm pain or tension so touch can feel good again. You deserve that support.

Some couples use sensate practice purely for connection, never making orgasm part of it, and they find that their intimacy still deepens like crazy. Others discover orgasms showing up as a surprise gift. Both stories are beautiful, and both are biblical. The experiences are yours to write.

PRACTICE 2. WORD PLAY

You already text flirty messages and emojis during the day. Think of this as the grown-up, naked version.

How to play:

1. One spouse lies face-down (or face-up once you're comfortable).
2. The other uses a fingertip, feather, fork tine, ice cube, or warm spoon to slowly trace a short word, phrase, or emoji on the back, butt, or inner thigh of the receiver.
3. The receiver guesses what was traced. Wrong guess equals another deliciously-slow trace.
4. Some idea phrases to start: "loved," "chosen," "wanted," "yummy," "best friend."
5. Some emoji ideas to start: heart, peach, the heart eye smiley face—use your imagination!
6. When the receiver guesses correctly, he or she gets to trace something back.

PRACTICE 3. HAND SKILLS

Did you get married and ever pull a Ricky Bobby in *Talladega Nights* and whisper in the dark, "I don't know what to do with my hands"? Still feel that way some nights? You're not alone. Many Christian couples have two perfectly good hands that only know two speeds: awkward grope or folded in prayer. Let's give those hands a confident upgrade.

Below is a menu of options. Every item works anywhere on the body. Don't worry: We'll tell you exactly how to use those hands on the erogenous zones, too. A lot of us never got the memo on how to touch the parts God made for pleasure. We give a lot of options here. Feel free to try them over a series of intimate encounters. There's no need to rush.

Flat-Palm Glide

Warm a little coconut oil or lube between your palms until it warms up. Lay both flat hands on your spouse's skin and make one long, continuous stroke. Think of smoothing frosting on a cake, except the cake is your spouse and the frosting is the moisturizer.

On erogenous zones: For her, cup the whole vulva gently in one warm palm and just hold for ten seconds (no movement yet). Then glide slowly upward over the mons pubis (check the anatomy pictures in Part 1 for reference) and back down. For him, wrap one flat-palm under the testicles and the other over the shaft and glide from base to tip in one slow motion. Repeat until they forget their own name—or say yours—repeatedly.

Fingertip Fireworks

Use only the soft pads of your fingertips. Move them in tiny random patterns so light it almost tickles—but doesn't quite. Picture a spider doing ballet on the skin.

On erogenous zones: Trace the outer labia as if you're drawing lazy infinity symbols. Circle the head of the penis with one fingertip, barely grazing the corona (that ridge where the head meets the shaft). Move to the inner labia for her or the underside of the penis near the head of the penis with the same feather touch. Goosebumps and hip twitches mean jackpot.

The Heartbeat Press

Place your whole palm over the heart and breathe with him or her for three counts. Then, without lifting your hand, slowly drag it straight down the centerline of the body, sternum to belly button. Pause and press gently but firmly as you glide. Observe what you and your spouse prefer: deep, firm pressure of the full hand? the more sweeping pressure of the flat-palm glide from earlier? Continue to observe what sensations you feel and how it feeds desire. Part of the thrill is communicating those observations!

On erogenous zones: Continue that same line all the way down. For her, end with your palm resting over the entire vulva, holding steady warmth; for him, let the hand keep traveling until your palm covers the shaft and your fingertips rest on the testicles. Some may find that from here they jump back to fingertip fireworks practice, or whatever touch you both communicate that feels good in that moment.

The Kneady Lover

The kneady lover is like kneading bread dough, but *way* more tenderly in the sacred spots. Grab a muscle group with your whole hand, squeeze gently, roll, release, move an inch, and repeat. This works wonders on tight necks, lower backs, and calves, but when you bring it downstairs, shift into a slower, silkier gear.

For him, inner thighs and butt cheeks love the classic knead (it brings blood flow and feels possessive in the best way). When you reach the testicles, though, imagine you're holding something far more precious than bread dough (like Gollum holding the One Ring, his "Precious"). Cup them lightly in one warm, oiled hand and roll them very gently between your fingers and palm, the same way those old Chinese Baoding stress balls used to clink and rotate smoothly in corporate guys' hands back in the nineties—no squeezing, just slow, continuous, weightless rolling. Most men melt and make a sound they didn't know they had in them.

For the shaft, switch to a loose, open-hand cradle: Rest it in your palm, close your fingers lightly around it, and rock or roll your hand in tiny motions so the skin glides over the erectile tissue underneath. Remember to keep gentle pressure here—or ask your husband if he wants a firmer hold.

For her, knead the inner thighs and butt exactly like warm dough, slowly, deliberately, and rhythmically. When you move to the more sensitive areas, soften everything. Cup the entire vulva in one warm palm and gently rock or roll your hand in tiny circles so the outer and inner labia move under your touch like silk under water. Alternate with the flat-palm glide so that she feels both held and teased. If she's aroused and swollen, you can use the same Baoding ball motion on the outer labia: lightly roll the tissue between thumb and fingers, never pinching, just luxurious, continuous movement. It's the feminine version of the testicle roll, and it usually produces the same wide-eyed, oh-my-goodness reaction.

Wherever you are on the body, if your spouse sighs more deeply, stay. If the body tenses, lighten up or move an inch away, or move away and come back later—unless you're told that it's a don't-stop kind of tension, in which case, keep going. The kneady lover is all about communicating, "I could do this for hours because every part of you is worthy of my attention."

The Swirl

One or two fingertips making tiny, slow circles the size of a dime is how the swirl works. Pick anywhere on the body and give it a try—neck, shoulder, chest, breasts, thighs, feet, hands. You get the point.

On erogenous zones: For her, begin beside the clitoris, never directly at first. For him, circle the hood or the shaft indirectly for a minute or two, then gradually move the circles closer. When arousal is obvious (swelling, wetness, or hardness), you may circle directly on the clitoral glans or the head of the penis, but keep it whisper-light at first. Ask, "More pressure or perfect?" and let the body and voice have a vote.

The Two-Finger (or Three-Finger) Slide

Warm lube on your fingers. Gently sandwich the body part between two fingers and glide up and down in one fluid motion. For her, start with the outer labia only. Once she's breathing faster, part the outer labia and glide along the inner labia, brushing past (but not entering) the vaginal opening. When she's clearly ready, let one finger glide over the clitoris on every upward stroke.

For him, sandwich the shaft between two fingers (or wrap all four if he likes more pressure). Glide root to tip, letting your thumb swirl the head on every upstroke. Occasionally pause at the base and gently tug downward to create delicious tension.

Golden Rules for the Whole Menu

- Always warm your hands first.
- Watch your spouse's body more than his or her face: deeper breath, arching, reaching for you, wetness, or hardness are all enthusiastic yeses.
- Laugh if it tickles.
- Ask simple questions: Harder? Softer? Faster? Slower? Right there?
- Sometimes, the best touch is the one that says, "I see all of you and I'm still here." That's the touch that heals and heats in the same moment.

Tonight, pick three techniques and spend five long minutes on each. By the end of the week, your hands will speak fluent Spouse, and Ricky Bobby will be officially retired from your bedroom.

PRACTICE 4. MOUTH SKILLS

Your mouth was made for more than casual conversations, kissing babies, and saying "amen" at the end of prayers. Breath, whisper, lips, tongue—every single part is welcome and celebrated in your marriage. God gave you taste buds, lips that can pout or smile, and a tongue that can speak truth and bring pleasure. Let's put them all to holy, playful use.

Start Here

This is your no-pressure progression. Begin with the safest, most-clothed spots and move toward erogenous zones only when both of you are nodding with excitement. Again, the goal is never about performance; it's more about, "I'm savoring you because you are a gift." Friendly reminder: Brushing your teeth and taking a shower are always recommended before placing your mouths all over one another. Also, you may want to cautious before putting a minty mouth down yonder—it may feel a little spicy. While we're at it, here's an overall hygiene reminder: It can get sweaty and—well—smelly after a full day of living life. If you think about what hits the brakes on desire and arousal, nothing hits the brakes quite like the smell of unleashed scrotum sweat. Please, take a shower. Also, communicate with your spouse about preferred scents for perfumes, soaps, shampoos, and so forth. Some individuals have aversions to certain smells or may even get headaches or nausea from scents.

Warm Breath Hover

Hover your mouth one to two inches from the skin (no contact yet) and exhale slowly, letting warm, moist breath wash over it. Prime spots on which to begin are at the back of the neck, ear (especially the outer edge and lobe), inner wrist, lower belly just above the waistband, and inner thigh (clothed or bare). Watch the body respond: hairs stand up, skin flushes, maybe a shiver or a sigh. These positive responses are your green light.

Whisper Truth

While still hovering, speak right against the skin so that the vibration of your voice adds another layer. Try these short phrases (or make up your own):

- "You are my favorite place to be."
- "I love the way you feel."
- "I want you right now."
- "Your skin tastes like home."
- "You make my heart race."
- "I can't get enough of you."

Whisper slowly, letting your lips brush the skin lightly as you speak. The combination of warm breath plus words plus vibration is electric.

Gentle Kisses That Build

Start with soft, closed-mouth kisses, light and lingering. Graduate to open-mouthed kisses. Let your lips part slightly, press more fully, linger longer. Then add the lightest graze of tongue—just the tip touching the skin for a split second, then pulling back.

Progression spots include the collarbone, shoulder, side of the neck, jawline, inner forearm, and belly button (circle it with your tongue if there's a giggle).

For Him: Shaft and Head

Start with soft, closed-mouthed kisses along the entire length of the shaft (base to tip) as if you're savoring every inch. Then progress to open-mouthed kisses, letting your lips slide over the skin. Swirl your tongue around the head. Start at the corona (that ridge), circle slowly with the tip of your tongue, and then flick the very tip lightly if he's moaning. Take the head into your mouth gently: warm, wet, and absolutely no teeth! Use your tongue to press and swirl while your lips create a soft seal. A variation is to hum softly while the head is in your mouth. The vibration feels incredible.

Once he's more firm, he may enjoy a quicker pace. You can take both his head and shaft fully into your mouth and move your head up and down while keeping a slight suction with your lips.

You can also cup the testicles in one hand and roll them gently (again, the Baoding balls) while you work the shaft with your mouth. Dual sensation heaven.

For Her: Inner Thighs to Clitoris Savoring

Begin with slow, open-mouthed kisses on the inner thighs. Start mid-thigh and work upward. You can do one leg and then the other, or you can alternate legs as you go. Kiss the crease where thigh meets vulva, then the outer labia.

Use long, slow licks. Start from the vaginal entrance and lick upward to the clitoris, using the flat of your tongue for broad coverage or the tip for more targeted strokes. Keep each lick deliberate and controlled. Once she's swollen and breathing hard, part the outer labia gently with your fingers and use the tip of your tongue to circle the clitoral hood first (indirect pressure). When she's clearly ready, approach direct contact: swirl the tongue around the glans (the exposed part of the clitoris), then flick lightly side-to-side or up-and-down.

As a variation, you can use gentle suction at the clitoris. Keep it gentle unless more pressure is requested. Another option is to draw the clitoris softly into your mouth while your tongue swirls. Alternate with slow licks to keep variety.

Try using your hands to knead the inner thighs or hold your wife's hips steady while you focus. If she's pregnant, postpartum, perimenopausal, or has sensitivity, you may want to stay broader and lighter and ask whether more or less pressure is desired.

RESPECTING BOUNDARIES WITH FINISHING

Oral play can feel incredibly intimate and generous, but it also brings up a very practical question: Where does he ejaculate? This is not something to leave to surprise or assumption. Every wife has her own comfort level, and those boundaries deserve full respect. No exceptions.

Have a calm, clothes-on conversation ahead of time (ideally not in the heat of the moment). Some wives are completely comfortable with finishing in the mouth. Many wives and husbands prefer that he finish on her chest, belly, thighs, a towel, during penetration, or by pulling away to use his own hand for the final strokes. Whatever you both agree to do is the right answer for your marriage.

If she says, "Not in my mouth," that boundary is loving, not rejecting. Honor it gladly and without pouting. Her trust and enthusiasm are worth it. Plan together where he will finish and keep a soft towel nearby for clean-up. When boundaries are clear and respected, both of you can relax and enjoy the moment without tension.

Mutual delight, never pressure, is always the goal. A husband who honors his wife's limits with care and respect often finds her more eager and playful in the long run. Respecting boundaries is a way to show your wife she is safe with you—and that hits the gas on her desire.

Golden Rules for Mouth Skills

- Consider warming your mouth (maybe sipping warm water if your lips and breath are not already warm). For some, cold breath is a mood killer. Others may like that cold sensation. Communicate preferences on mouth temperature if you have them.
- Don't use teeth unless specifically asked (and even then, use gentle nibbles only).
- Watch body language: Deeper breaths, hips lifting, and hands in your hair are often signs to keep going. Pulling away or tensing often means you should lighten up or move elsewhere. If you're not sure what the body language is communicating, just ask. Seriously. Communication of likes and dislikes is vital in the bedroom.
- Ask questions: Harder? Softer? Faster? Slower? Right here?
- If saliva builds up, that's normal and actually helpful for lubrication. Swallow or wipe discreetly if needed.
- Laugh if it gets messy. Messy is part of the fun.

It can be best to not try all of these mouth skills at once. For example, tonight, spend five minutes on breath and whispers and five minutes on kisses. Tomorrow, add one technique or swap out another technique, if you're both ready. Maybe it feels best to just try one to two minutes at first.

Your mouth is a gift and using it to adore your spouse is one of the sweetest ways to say, "I love you," without words.

PRACTICE 5. GROUNDING PRACTICE

Grounding practice is great for when your brain is spiraling but your body still longs to connect.

Some nights, the to-do list won't stop, the baby won't sleep, the sermon prep is looming, or anxiety just shows up uninvited. You're exhausted and overwhelmed, and the idea of "normal" intimacy feels like one more demand. Yet somewhere underneath, you still want to feel close to the person you love most. This grounding practice is for those nights. It meets you exactly where you are, clothes on, no pressure, and gently brings your mind, body, and soul back into the same room. Here's how to do it:

1. **Find a quiet spot and get comfortable together.** Sit facing each other on the bed, cross-legged or knees touching, or lie side-by-side if sitting feels too intense. Keep all clothes on for now. Dim the lights or keep one small lamp on—whatever helps you feel safe, not exposed.

2. **Connect hand to heart.** Both of you, place your right hand gently over your spouse's heart (right in the center of the chest). Let your left hands find each other and interlace fingers. Close your eyes if that helps you tune in, or keep soft eye contact if that feels more connecting tonight. Some people feel uncomfortable placing hands on hearts. If that's you, you can place both hands between your laps with fingers interlaced.

3. **Breathe together for two full minutes.** Inhale slowly through the nose for a count of four. Hold gently for a count of four. Exhale through the mouth for a count of six. Let your bellies rise and fall. Feel the warmth of your hands on your spouse and his or her hands on you. If your mind wanders (it will), just notice and come back to the next breath. You can set a quiet timer or count breaths. Ten to twelve deep, calming breaths last about two minutes.

4. **Ground your senses together.** Still holding hands to hearts, take turns naming the following (out loud or silently, whichever feels better):
   - Three things you can see right now (even with eyes closed: the glow behind your eyelids, the outline of the face, the color of the sheets).
   - Two things you feel on your skin (the weight of the hand, the softness of the blanket, the air on your face).
   - One thing you're thankful for about the person in front of you ("I'm thankful you're here with me tonight," "I'm thankful for the way you love our kids," "I'm thankful your heart is still beating under my hand"). No need to elaborate, just name it simply and sincerely.

5. **Check in about clothes and next steps.** After the breathing and grounding, pause and ask quietly, "Do you want to stay just like this, or would taking off a layer feel good?" Undress only as far as feels safe and inviting. Maybe it's just removing socks, maybe shirts, maybe nothing at all tonight. There is no wrong answer.

6. **Return to hands on hearts and add slow, present touch.** Come back to the same hand-to-heart position (or shift to spooning if that feels better). Keep the same slow breathing rhythm. Begin to add simple, no-goal

caresses: trace your spouse's arm with your free hand, stroke hair, or rub slow circles on the back. Stay present. Notice texture, warmth, and the rise and fall of the breath under your palm. If arousal stirs, let it come naturally. If tears come instead, let those come naturally too.

7. **Let whatever happens next be enough.** Some nights, you'll drift into deeper touch and lovemaking. Some nights, you'll fall asleep still holding one another. Some nights, one of you will pray out loud while the other just listens. All of it is connected. All of it is worship. All of it counts.

Note. Do not pressure your spouse into sex—*ever.* Caressing and cuddling should only lead to more if both spouses agree to it. If one of you feels complete with a certain step, honor that boundary with gratitude, not disappointment. Caressing, cuddling, or any step forward should only continue if both of you joyfully agree. That means no coaxing, no guilt, no subtle pushing. Scripture reminds us, "Daughters of Jerusalem, I charge you . . . Do not arouse or awaken love until it so desires" (Song of Songs 2:7). When a spouse says, "This is enough for tonight," it is not rejection; your spouse is trusting you with his or her heart. Receive that trust as sacred, respond with tenderness, and watch how such safety can open the door wider as love and trust deepen and grow.

Grounding practice reminds your nervous system that touch can be safe; it reminds your heart that your spouse is for you; and it reminds your soul that God is right there in the quiet with you both. Some couples may make this something they do as a regular part of their connection rhythm, even on good nights, as they discover how it takes them from overwhelmed to open again.

PRACTICE 6. PROPS, PILLOWS, AND POSITIONS

We get the following question a lot: Are sex toys or props okay for Christians? Here's the simple truth: The Bible celebrates intimacy in marriage as a good gift and never speaks against tools or toys that help couples enjoy that gift with more comfort, pleasure, or connection. Anything mutually loving, respectful, and agreed upon together falls well within the freedom God gives husbands and wives. It is important to talk it over with your spouse first to find out what you may or may not feel comfortable with. You should never force toys (or anything) into the equation when someone feels uncomfortable.

Pillows Are the MVP (and the Easiest Place to Start)

A few ordinary pillows (or one firm one) can change everything about comfort and sensation. They support tired bodies, shift angles for better access, and can help remove pain. Here are a few ideas on how to use pillows:

Wife on Her Back, Pillow under Hips

This gentle tilt can allow for different sensory-rich areas of the vagina to experience pleasure during penetration and makes clitoral stimulation easier for both partners. It also takes strain off the neck during oral sex, letting you linger longer without ache.

Prone (Facedown) with a Pillow or Two under Her Pelvis

The slight lift allows deeper penetration while keeping her back flat and relaxed. Many couples find this position eliminates lower-back pain when approaching from this angle. Some people find a wedge pillow to be nice in this same position with the hips resting on the taller portion of the wedge and the chest resting on the narrower portion of the wedge pillow. You can also use a few pillows under the hips and one under the chest if you don't have access to a wedge pillow.

Side-Lying Spoon with Pillow between Knees

This keeps hips aligned and reduces pressure on the lower back or pelvis. It can be pure gold postpartum or anytime one of you needs gentle, close connection without weight or strain.

Positions for Pain or Discomfort

Small shifts can make intimacy possible again when bodies are sore, healing, or changing. Here are a few position options for when you or your spouse is experiencing pain or discomfort:

Chronic Hip Pain

Try the pretzel (one partner lies on the side, the other kneels and straddles the bottom leg while holding the top leg up) or seated on a sturdy chair facing each other. Both keep hips in a neutral, open position.

Low-Back Pain

Let the wife sit on top (she controls depth and speed) or use hands-and-knees with pillows stacked under her chest and belly for full support. These options take some pressure off the spine.

Pelvic Floor Tension or Pain

Start together in child's pose (kneeling, hips back toward heels, forehead down, husband approaching from behind) and simply breathe and rock gently. From there you can transition slowly to side-lying or missionary (face-to-face with one partner on top with plenty of pillows under knees and low back). In missionary position with the husband on top, having pillows on the sides of the wife's legs holding her legs up so that she can fully relax her legs instead of holding them up on her own can also help relieve pelvic floor tension and pain.

Props We Love

These props are simple, non-intimidating additions that enhance pleasure without ever becoming the focus. The focus always stays on each other.

- **Blindfolds:** Using a blindfold heightens every other sense and builds trust as you rely on touch, breath, and voice alone.
- **Wedge pillows:** Wedge pillows can be store-bought, such as Liberator shapes, or homemade with stacked pillows. They give the same reliable lift as regular pillows but stay put so you never have to pause and readjust.
- **Vibrators:** We cover these fully in Practice 9, but for now know they're simply tools for adding sensation, just like hands or mouths.
- **Feather ticklers, silk scarves for gentle tying, or warmed coconut oil for massage:** Song of Songs is full of scented oils, spices, and playful delight. These items bring that same spirit of lavish, sensory adoration into your bedroom today.

If anyone ever worries about "misusing the body" (which is misquoting 1 Corinthians 6:19, by the way), gently point out that the verse right before it celebrates the beautiful mystery of two becoming one. Tools that help you unite with more joy, comfort, and closeness honor that mystery, not violate it.

Start with pillows tonight. They are already in your house, cost nothing, and can transform an ordinary night into one you both remember with smiles. From there, add whatever props spark mutual curiosity and gratitude. Your marriage bed is honored and undefiled (Hebrews 13:4). Make it as comfortable and delightful as God allows.

PRACTICE 7. SENSORY PLAY

God wired us with five glorious senses, and He didn't leave them at the bedroom door. Sight, sound, smell, taste, and touch were all part of His "very good" design from the beginning. When we bring them intentionally into intimacy, something ordinary becomes extraordinary. The same bodies you've known for years suddenly feel new, alive, and worth cherishing. Sensory play isn't about adding complexity; it's about noticing the details God already put there and saying thank You with your whole self.

Try these gentle, playful ways to wake up each sense. Pick one or two to start (no need to do all five every time). The goal is to develop awareness and to learn how to enjoy the pleasure of fully engaging your senses intimately with your spouse. This practice is not a checklist.

Sight

Turn the lights low with a bedside lamp or scatter a few candles for a soft, flickering glow. Many couples love placing a mirror where you can catch glimpses of each other; watching your spouse's face or body respond to your touch can feel vulnerably beautiful and deeply connecting. If mirrors feel too intense at first, just keep eye contact longer than usual and notice the color of the eyes in this light. Let yourself be aware of what your eyes take in and delight in it.

Sound

Create a shared playlist of songs that mean something to your story (maybe pull up the one from when you were dating)—or skip the music entirely and listen to the symphony you make together: the catch of breath, the soft moan, the contented sigh, the whispered "yes" or "I love you." Paying attention to those sounds turns them into feedback that guides you both closer.

Smell

Dab a drop of essential oil on pulse points (wrists, neck, behind ears). Ylang-ylang, sweet orange, or cedarwood are naturally calming and sensual, but your favorite shared scent works even better (the cologne he wore on your wedding day or the lotion she loves). Scent ties straight to memory and emotion, so one whiff can pull you both right back to honeymoon feelings or quiet gratitude for the years since. Again, just another friendly reminder to shower. While smell can be a turn on, it can also be a hard turn off. I know we keep mentioning it, but the amount of times Kelsey has been told by clients that one spouse's lack of hygiene is one of the biggest hurdles in their sex life will never cease to amaze us.

Taste

Bring something simple and fun to bed: chocolate-dipped strawberries, chilled grapes, a square of dark chocolate, or even a warm or cool beverage—or keep it beautifully basic and taste your spouse's skin right after a shower, noticing the clean warmth of the neck, shoulder, or inner wrist. Taste reminds you that your spouse is someone to savor, not rush. Friendly reminder: Nothing flavored or scented goes in the vagina. No one wants to throw off the pH balance and get vaginal irritation or a yeast infection.

Touch

Pull from everything we've already covered (and more): Drag a feather slowly across skin, trail an ice cube followed by warm breath, massage with warmed coconut oil, let silk scarves glide over curves, or (if you're feeling spicy) try a Wartenberg wheel for that (gentle!) tingly pinpoint sensation. The Wartenberg wheel, a handheld metal tool with a rotating spiked wheel, and other tools often used in the rehabilitation therapy and massage therapy worlds (that you can find at retail stores) can feel like a whole new world of tactile sensation to explore in the bedroom. Things like a spiked massage ball, trigger point release ball, palm massage tool, and massage roller balls are often things we consider for pain relief, but they can also be used for pleasurable foreplay or even as the main event.

Create Variety

A key to deepening pleasure can mean creating variety, for example, alternating light and firm, cool and warm, ticklish and deep. Touch is the sense we use most in intimacy, so waking it up with contrast makes every caress feel brand new.

Start with whichever sense feels easiest. It can be great to focus on or high-light just one sense for the experience even though all are involved. You can also layer them together (candles for sight, playlist for sound, scented oil for smell) and watch how your bedroom becomes a place where the whole you shows up: mind awake, body alive, and soul grateful. This is the kind of play that leaves you both smiling, closer, and whispering, "This is good," long after the candles burn out.

PRACTICE 8. DESIRE BUILDERS (THROUGHOUT THE DAY AND IN THE BEDROOM)

Desire isn't a light switch you flip on at bedtime. It's a fire you tend all day with small, steady acts of attention and affection. Those little moments remind your spouse, "I see you, I want you, I'm glad you're mine," and they turn everyday life into the runway for joyful intimacy later.

Daily Deposits

A daily deposit is a small, intentional act of connection done consistently over time. It's not about grand gestures or perfect moments, but about choosing regular, low-pressure ways to show care, attention, and presence. Those small moments quietly build trust, safety, and closeness from which intimacy grows. Pick one to try. They're simple, but they add up.

Send One Specific Appreciation Text a Day

Make it pointed: "Still thinking about your shoulders in that shirt this morning," or "The way you laughed at dinner replayed in my head all afternoon," or "The way you handled that toddler meltdown was ridiculously attractive." Specificity makes your spouse feel truly seen, and that feeling is rocket fuel for desire.

Five-Second Hugs with Deep Eye Contact

Do five-second hugs with deep eye contact when you wake up, when one comes home, and before bed. The oxytocin boost is real, but the real magic is remembering that your spouse is your home.

Leave a Flirty Post-It Note

You can put a note on the bathroom mirror, coffee mug, or dashboard. Examples include "Tonight you're mine" or just a heart and a wink.

In the Bedroom

Take those deposits of desire you've made throughout the day and take them to the bedroom.

The Ten-Minute Make-Out Session

Kiss deeply for ten full minutes, hands over clothes, no rushing further. Some nights you stop there and fall asleep smiling. The nights you don't? Well, that's great, too. Be sure to communicate one another's experiences, desires, and preferences with consideration and respect.

Read Song of Songs 7

Read Song of Songs 7 out loud to each other as if it's foreplay—because it is. Take turns, slowly letting the words land. Touch what's being described if it feels natural. God's poetry gives you permission to speak beauty over each other's bodies.

For Hard Seasons

When you are a caregiver (to your kids, your parents), schedules are brutal, or desire feels low for medical reasons, you may need to scale daily deposits down or scale them up. Find ways to connect that meet your needs where you are at and communicate those needs with your spouse. A single text and one long hug still count. A whispered "I'm thankful for you" while passing in the hallway still builds. God honors the small offerings, and over time they add up to renewed hunger.

Start with one daily deposit this week. Watch how the little things you do outside of the bedroom can make your relationship more intimate—and connected.

PRACTICE 9. CAN WE VIBE?

Let's say it plainly: Vibrators are allowed in your bedroom. If you ask us for a verse to support it, well, that's going to be hard to do because vibrators didn't exist when the Bible was written—along with a whole variety of things we use today that serve as tools and aids to help us relax and feel pleasure: massage chairs, modern-day mattresses and pillows, hot tubs, and more. That's right. It's okay to pause a moment and thank God for some modern inventions.

Here's what we do know. God created thousands of nerve endings that respond beautifully to steady rhythmic pressure, and modern tools simply deliver that sensation more consistently than fingers, hands, or mouths sometimes can. They are not a replacement for your spouse; they are optional helpers that can make good things even better, especially when fatigue, postpartum changes, menopause, or other seasons can make arousal harder to come by. Used with mutual enthusiasm and gratitude, they can be used to honor the bodies God gave you both.

If you've never used a vibrator before—no worries!—you're just starting a new adventure together. Take it slow, laugh a lot, and keep talking. Below, you will find some helpful information on types of vibrators and tips to help build your confidence with using them. Feel free to start with whichever type of vibrator feels least intimidating.

Bullet

Small, discreet, and often lipstick-sized, these are great for pinpoint stimulation on the clitoris, nipples, or perineum (the sensitive area between vulva or testicles and the anus). Easy to hold and control, bullet vibrators can be a great place to start for beginners.

Wand

Wand vibrators are larger, with a big, rounded head and serious power. There are many compact, waterproof, and chargeable options out there for wands. Some are corded. We recommend getting a chargeable, cordless option because the corded versions are restrictive for positioning and literally tie you to an outlet. Wands can be amazing for back, shoulder, or thigh massages and can also be used for clitoral stimulation. The broad head spreads vibration, so it usually doesn't feel too intense at first on the lower settings.

Egg

Slightly larger and oval-shaped, egg vibrators often come with a retrieval string. They are designed for insertion vaginally for internal pressure and pleasure, but many couples use them externally too. They're usually whisper-quiet and often remote or app controlled for playful teasing.

Suction (or Air Pulse)

Suction vibrators don't vibrate in the traditional way; instead, they use gentle air pulses or suction to surround the clitoris without direct contact. Many women describe it as feeling like oral sex. The sensation can feel intense but indirect. Some of these vibrators include traditional vibration with the air pulsing. Popular options include rose-style or smaller vibrators with a nozzle. They can be great for clitoral focus without the numbness that some get with wand use.

Therapeutic Options

Therapeutic options are especially helpful if pain, tightness, or pelvic floor tension is part of your story. (If you are experiencing any pain, tension, discomfort, please see a pelvic health occupational or physical therapist for help.)

Kiwi

A Kiwi, from The Pelvic People, is a multi-end vibrating massager created specifically for pelvic floor relaxation and entry pain relief. It has gentle shapes for external massage (thighs, perineum, clitoris), shallow internal use, and deeper muscle release. Vibration helps increase blood flow, desensitize tender areas, and build positive touch associations. Many couples find it bridges therapy and pleasure beautifully.

Vibrating Pelvic Wand

This long, curved, medical-grade silicone wand has multiple vibration speeds. It was designed by pelvic health therapists for trigger point release inside the vagina or rectum, perineal massage, and relaxing deep pelvic muscles. It was initially designed as a clinical tool (great for postpartum healing or chronic tension), and many couples have found it useful for intimate play as well.

These therapeutic styles of vibrators are often recommended by pelvic health professionals because vibration promotes increased blood circulation, helps relax overactive muscles, and can make intimacy possible again when pain and tension have been a barrier.

How to Use Vibrators

Unbox and Prepare Your Vibrator

Fully charge your vibrator. Wash with mild, unscented soap and water or spray toy cleaner. Have a towel nearby and your favorite lube ready. Turn it on in your hand first, away from skin, to feel the different speeds and patterns. Remember not to take yourself too seriously with this. It's okay to laugh at the funny buzz sound!

Start on the Least Intimidating Spot of Your Body

If it feels better for you, keep your clothes on at first. Use the lowest speed and press gently against your spouse's shoulders, neck, lower back, feet, or outer thighs. Treat the vibrator like a fancy massage tool—which is essentially what it is. Notice how the vibration travels through muscle and relaxes tension. Spend five or ten minutes here just getting comfortable with the feeling.

Progress Slowly to More Sensitive Areas

When you're both feeling ready, move to the bikini line, inner thighs, base of the penis, or outer labia (still over underwear if you want). Start by using broad pressure, not pinpoint yet. Let the receiver guide the direction: "A little higher," "Slower," "Right there." The giver's other hand can stay connected by holding a hand or stroking hair to keep progress relational. It could be that you are both the giver and the receiver in the sense that you are holding the vibrator and using it on your own body to get to know what it feels like before guiding your spouse on how to use it with you. For some, they prefer to always be the one holding the vibrator while using it on themselves, and that's okay, too.

Introduce Clitoral or Penile Stimulation

For her, start with the broad side or lowest setting over the clitoral hood (never straight on the glans at first—that can be too intense). Move in slow circles or side-to-side. Once arousal builds (think swelling and wetness), you can use the tip for more focused pressure or increase the speed slightly. For suction-style vibrators, center the nozzle over the clitoris and let the air pulses do the work. Start on the gentlest setting.

For him, press gently along the shaft, under the head, or on the perineum. Many men love steady vibration at the underside of the penis near the head or at the base or the penis during manual or oral play. One of you may prefer a more intense setting than the other. You may want to start off on a gentler setting and then increase in intensity as arousal builds.

Keep the Speed on Low to Start during Intercourse

Place the toy where it adds sensation without overwhelming: on her clitoris, his perineum, or against the base of the penis. A bullet, wand, or suction toy held by either partner works. Move slowly as you are learning the new sensations. Vibration amplifies everything, so less thrusting is often more when using a vibrator when the penis is in the vagina. Check in often: Too much? Perfect? Want to pause? As always, communication is key.

Lube and Care Rules

Use water-based lubricant generously with any silicone vibrator (silicone lube can degrade the material). With non-silicone toys you have more options, but water-based lube is always safe and easy to clean. After play, wash the vibrator immediately with warm water and mild unscented soap, dry thoroughly, and store in its pouch away from other toys. There are also unscented mild adult toy spray cleaners that are a convenient way to clean vibrators.

Golden Rules for Vibrator Use

- Vibrator use should always include a mutual yes. Never surprise someone with a vibrator. You should talk about it first.
- Keep communicating: "Show me where," "Tell me when to stop," "That feels amazing."
- If the vibration feels weird or too intense, turn off the vibrator and go back to hands and mouths. Doing so is not failure; it is listening to and respecting what is best for you.
- Start with the vibrator of your choice on a relaxed, no-pressure night. Use it for massage first, then let curiosity lead the way. You might discover new favorite sensations, easier orgasms, or just a lot of giggles. All of it is good, all of it is allowed, and all of it can draw you closer in mind, body, and soul.

PRACTICE 10. THE SLOW BUILD

Some days call for quick connection, and that's a gift too. But other days (date nights, anniversaries, or "we finally have the house to ourselves") are made for lingering. The slow build is about turning forty-five to ninety minutes into deliberate, escalating pleasure with no rushing. You savor every course, let anticipation do its work, and discover that delaying the peak often makes the peak higher than you thought possible. This practice teaches control, deepens trust, and reminds you both that your bodies were designed for wonder, not just efficiency.

Set the Stage

Lock the door, silence phones, dim lights, and put on quiet music or none at all. Have warmed oil, lube, towels, and water nearby. Agree up front: Tonight is about the journey, not a race to the finish. If kids wake up or life interrupts, laugh, pause the clock, and pick up again later. No pressure.

Roadmap

This roadmap is a flexible guide designed to help you slow down, build arousal gradually, and stay connected to each other throughout a dedicated forty-five-to-ninety-minute experience. Feel free to mix and match the activities below. You can even repeat the activities that are your favorites.

Ten-Minute Full-Body Massage Each

Yes, this means twenty full minutes touching one another's bodies. Warm coconut oil or your favorite massage oil or lotion between your palms—unless your spouse enjoys the cold feeling fresh out of the bottle, then by all means, put the oil or lotion directly on your spouse before warming it in your hands first. Check with one another to find out what the preferences are. Next, one spouse lies face-down. Spend five slow minutes on the back, shoulders, arms, buttocks, and legs. Flip over and do five minutes on the chest, belly, thighs, and feet without focusing on genitals or spending the entire five minutes on the breasts—because we know some of you will try.

Then switch roles. Keep the focus on connection and building a sense of awe for one another. Breathe together, notice every curve and scar, and whisper gratitude for the body under your hands. This alone builds arousal quietly and helps relax tensions that hurried sex usually ignores.

Ten Minutes Oral or Manual Only (Still No Penetration)

Choose who receives first. The giver uses everything you've learned: hands skills from Practice 3, mouth skills from Practice 4, maybe a toy from Practice 9. Focus on building heat slowly: long licks, gentle swirls, and full-palm glides.

The receiver's job is breathe, notice, and enjoy. No directing the giver to "finish me." If arousal climbs fast, say "slow down" or "pause." The goal is warm, buzzing pleasure, not orgasm—yet.

Edging: Bring Almost to Orgasm, Back Off, Repeat Three to Five Times

Edging is the secret sauce of extended pleasure. Continue oral, manual, or toy play until the receiver feels the unmistakable climb toward orgasm (muscles tighten, breath quickens, hips lift). Right before the point of no return, stop all stimulation for twenty to sixty seconds. Kiss, hold, breathe together, whisper something sweet ("You are stunning like this"). Repeat the cycle three to five times. Each peak gets higher, each valley deeper. Men learn ejaculatory control; women often discover multiple waves or stronger full-body orgasms. It teaches trust ("I can let go, and you'll still be here") and builds to final intensity.

When You Finally Join, Go Slowly

Penetration happens only when both of you are practically begging. Start with a shallow, gentle entry. Do ten achingly slow strokes. Count them out loud if you want. Then pause fully inside, kiss deeply, look into each other's eyes.

Repeat the cycle: Ten slow strokes, pause, connect. As you go, it's okay if you stop counting strokes.

For variation, stay still inside for moments and let her pelvic floor pulse around him, or rock gently without thrusting. Add clitoral or perineal vibration on low if you like. The slowness feels torturous at first, then transcendent.

Finish with simultaneous orgasm if you'd like and can, or you can take turns. When you sense the final climb, it's okay to ask, "Together or you first?" Simultaneous release is great when it happens naturally, but it shouldn't be forced, and there shouldn't be pressure to perform. More often, one partner goes over the edge first while the other holds and adores, then the roles reverse. Ideally you don't leave your spouse hanging. Either way, stay connected afterward. Breathe together, hold hands, snuggle, spoon—do whatever feels right in that moment that the two of you agree upon and communicate to one another. Thank God out loud for the gift you just shared. Let aftershocks and laughter roll through you.

MIX AND MATCHING THE PRACTICES

Here's the best part: None of these ten practices are meant to live in isolation. Think of them more as ingredients in your favorite recipe. You grab whatever sounds good tonight, toss in a pinch of this and a dash of that, and create something wonderfully yours.

For example, your choice for the evening may be penetrative intimacy as the main course, and everything else as the sides and seasonings you fold right in. While joined, you can keep tracing slow sensual circles on a back or thigh, whispering word-play against an ear, or telling your spouse exactly how much you're enjoying sex ("more," "harder," "mmm, yes!") between breaths. Your hands may be staying busy with Practice 3: swirls around nipples, heartbeat presses down the chest, or gentle kneading of inner thighs. Mouths don't clock out either: soft kisses along the neck, warm breath on skin, or the occasional long slow lick in reachable spots.

Pillows stay under hips or knees for perfect angles and zero pain. Sensory play keeps the atmosphere alive. You take in the scented oil still on skin, low candlelight flickering, and your shared playlist humming quietly. If anxiety creeps in or something feels momentarily off, slip into a quick grounding breath together, communicating if you need to slow down, change positions, or pull out. The desire you built all day with texts and hugs now fuels every movement. A gentle vibrator on low can rest against her clitoris or his perineum, adding shared hum without stealing center stage.

Sometimes you'll pull from two practices. Some nights you'll weave five. Some nights you'll stick to one favorite and let it shine. There's no perfect combination, only the one that makes you both sigh, laugh, and feel closer to each other and to God. Experiment, talk about what felt amazing, tweak what didn't, and keep playing. Your bedroom is a playground, not a stage. Mix, match, and make these practices your own. Over the years, we have seen that the couple who plays together, communicates together, and prays together gets to enjoy this gift for decades to come.

LET'S CHECK BACK IN: THE CONNECTED INTIMACY CHECK-IN

Hey, look! You made it to the end! Let's reflect a little before closing this book. We invite you to complete the Connected Intimacy Check-In again. This is the same reflection you completed earlier, and you are taking it a second time on purpose. The goal is to notice what has shifted as you have moved through this book together. Some areas may feel stronger. Some may feel unchanged. Others may feel newly tender because you now have language for things you could not see before. All of that is information, not failure.

As you answer these questions again, respond honestly based on how things feel right now. Let this second check-in help you recognize growth, name ongoing needs, and identify which practices or conversations you want to continue. Intimacy is not something you complete. It is something you return to, tend, and grow into over time, often with patience, grace, and support along the way.

Instructions

This check-in is included twice, once for each spouse. Complete your own version individually before discussing it together. Answer based on how things feel right now, not how you wish they felt or how they used to feel.

Rate each statement using the following scale:

0 Not true at all

1 Rarely true

2 Sometimes true

3 Often true

4 Very true

There are no right or wrong answers. You're obtaining information, not getting a grade.

Check-In 1

Category 1. Safety and being on the same team

1. I feel emotionally safe bringing up concerns about intimacy with my spouse.
2. I believe my spouse wants to understand my experience, even when it differs from his or hers.

3. We approach intimacy challenges as a shared issue rather than blaming one another.
4. I feel valued and cared for by my spouse outside of sexual moments.
5. When intimacy feels difficult, I trust we are still on the same team.

Category 2. Talking about intimacy with skill and grace

6. I have language to describe what I enjoy, do not enjoy, or feel unsure about sexually.
7. I feel able to say "no," "not right now," or "I need something different" without fear of consequences.
8. I feel comfortable initiating intimacy in ways that feel authentic to me.
9. We check in about intimacy rather than assuming the other person should know what we want.
10. Conversations about sex feel more curious than tense or avoidant.

Category 3. Desire, arousal, and honoring the body

11. I understand that desire does not always appear spontaneously and that this is normal.
12. I can identify personal factors that increase my openness to intimacy.
13. I can identify personal factors that decrease my openness to intimacy.
14. Physical factors such as stress, fatigue, pain, hormones, or health are acknowledged when we talk about intimacy.
15. Our approach to intimacy adapts to our bodies and seasons of life.

Category 4. Integrating mind, body, and soul

16. My faith feels integrated with intimacy rather than in conflict with it.
17. I believe pleasure and connection in marriage are good, meaningful, and something we both experience.
18. Shame does not dominate how I think about sex, my body, or my desires.
19. I feel free to bring my whole self into intimacy without fear or performance pressure.
20. Our shared values around intimacy feel life-giving rather than restrictive.

Category 5. Connected intimacy and growth over time

21. When intimacy does not go as planned, we are able to have a shame-free conversation about it and reconnect.
22. We can talk about disappointment or unmet expectations without withdrawing.
23. I feel hopeful that our intimacy can grow and change over time.
24. We approach intimacy as something we learn and practice, not something we should already know.
25. Intimacy feels like a shared journey rather than a problem to solve.

How to Score

- Rather than adding up all twenty-five questions, you will score each section separately. This helps you see where connection feels strong and where more attention may be helpful, without collapsing everything into a single number.
- Each section has five questions. Add your ratings for those five questions to get a section score.
- Each section score will fall between 0 and 20.

How to Interpret

Use the same interpretation scale for every section.

16–20

This area is currently a strength. It does not mean it is perfect, but it is likely supporting intimacy rather than blocking it. Maintain what is working and use it to support growth in other areas.

11–15

This area has a foundation with some tender spots. You may notice inconsistency or specific situations in which connection feels harder. Focus on the conversations and practices in the book that address this section.

6–10

This area likely needs attention with intent. Challenges here may be contributing to frustration, avoidance, or misunderstanding. This is a good place to slow down, to be curious, and to prioritize learning and practice. Outside help may be an option to consider.

0–5
This area feels strained or unsafe right now. This does not mean intimacy is broken or hopeless. Unresolved pain, unmet needs, or missing support may need to be addressed—perhaps by a professional. Extra care, patience, and outside help may be important here.

Reflection Questions
Which answers shifted, even slightly?

____

____

____

What new language or understanding do I have now?

____

____

____

What feels safer or easier to talk about than before?

____

____

____

What practices do we want to continue moving forward?

____

____

____

Check-In 2

Rate each statement using the following scale:
   5 Not true at all
   6 Rarely true

7 Sometimes true

8 Often true

9 Very true

There are no right or wrong answers. You're obtaining information, not getting a grade.

Category 1. Safety and being on the same team

6. I feel emotionally safe bringing up concerns about intimacy with my spouse.
7. I believe my spouse wants to understand my experience, even when it differs from his or hers.
8. We approach intimacy challenges as a shared issue rather than blaming one another.
9. I feel valued and cared for by my spouse outside of sexual moments.
10. When intimacy feels difficult, I trust we are still on the same team.

Category 2. Talking about intimacy with skill and grace

11. I have language to describe what I enjoy, do not enjoy, or feel unsure about sexually.
12. I feel able to say "no," "not right now," or "I need something different" without fear of consequences.
13. I feel comfortable initiating intimacy in ways that feel authentic to me.
14. We check in about intimacy rather than assuming the other person should know what we want.
15. Conversations about sex feel more curious than tense or avoidant.

Category 3. Desire, arousal, and honoring the body

16. I understand that desire does not always appear spontaneously and that this is normal.
17. I can identify personal factors that increase my openness to intimacy.
18. I can identify personal factors that decrease my openness to intimacy.
19. Physical factors such as stress, fatigue, pain, hormones, or health are acknowledged when we talk about intimacy.
20. Our approach to intimacy adapts to our bodies and seasons of life.

Category 4. Integrating mind, body, and soul

21. My faith feels integrated with intimacy rather than in conflict with it.
22. I believe pleasure and connection in marriage are good, meaningful, and something we both experience.
23. Shame does not dominate how I think about sex, my body, or my desires.
24. I feel free to bring my whole self into intimacy without fear or performance pressure.
25. Our shared values around intimacy feel life-giving rather than restrictive.

Category 5. Connected intimacy and growth over time

26. When intimacy does not go as planned, we are able to have a shame-free conversation about it and reconnect.
27. We can talk about disappointment or unmet expectations without withdrawing.
28. I feel hopeful that our intimacy can grow and change over time.
29. We approach intimacy as something we learn and practice, not something we should already know.
30. Intimacy feels like a shared journey rather than a problem to solve.

How to Score

- Rather than adding up all twenty-five questions, you will score each section separately. This helps you see where connection feels strong and where more attention may be helpful, without collapsing everything into a single number.
- Each section has five questions. Add your ratings for those five questions to get a section score.
- Each section score will fall between 0 and 20.

How to Interpret

Use the same interpretation scale for every section.

16–20

This area is currently a strength. It does not mean it is perfect, but it is likely supporting intimacy rather than blocking it. Maintain what is working and use it to support growth in other areas.

11–15

This area has a foundation with some tender spots. You may notice inconsistency or specific situations in which connection feels harder. Focus on the conversations and practices in the book that address this section.

6–10

This area likely needs attention with intent. Challenges here may be contributing to frustration, avoidance, or misunderstanding. This is a good place to slow down, to be curious, and to prioritize learning and practice. Outside help may be an option to consider.

0–5

This area feels strained or unsafe right now. This does not mean intimacy is broken or hopeless. Unresolved pain, unmet needs, or missing support may need to be addressed—perhaps by a professional. Extra care, patience, and outside help may be important here.

Reflection Questions

Which answers shifted, even slightly?

____

____

____

What new language or understanding do I have now?

____

____

____

What feels safer or easier to talk about than before?

____

____

____

What practices do we want to continue moving forward?

____

____

____

As you finish answering these questions, take a step back and reflect on how you've grown. Our bet is that the relationship you started this guide with is not the same one you are ending it with. You paid attention to yourself and to one another. You listened. You learned language for things that may have once felt confusing, awkward, or even forbidden. You noticed where intimacy feels strong and where it still needs care. That alone is meaningful work.

This guide was never meant to give you a checklist to complete or a finish line to cross. Relationships simply do not work this way. If you are waiting to feel like you've arrived, we hate to disappoint you, but you'll be waiting for a very long time. This guide was meant to invite you into a deeper way of seeing each other, your bodies, and your marriage. If some areas feel stronger now, give thanks. If some still feel tender, hold them with patience and hope. Growth does not require everything to be resolved. It requires willingness, humility, and love.

What follows next is not a summary of what you should do next, but a blessing over what you have already begun—a reminder of the holiness of your marriage, the goodness of embodied intimacy, and the joy God takes in your connection.

A BENEDICTION FOR YOUR MARRIAGE

You did it. You opened a book that many Christian couples never dare to open. You learned the actual names and wonders of the bodies God gave you. Yes, we're talking about the vulva, clitoris, pelvic floor, erectile tissue, and all. You discovered how arousal, desire, lubrication, and orgasm actually work, not from rumors or awkward youth-group talks, but from Scripture-honoring, evidence-based truth.

You sat together for ten brave conversations. You talked about common issues that quietly steal joy: mismatched desire, body image struggles after babies, past wounds, performance pressure, exhaustion, shame from bad teaching, and the fear that "good Christians" aren't supposed to want this much. You laughed, you blushed, and maybe you cried, but you spoke truth in love and listened with grace.

Then you put what you learned into practice. You rediscovered touch with sensate focus, learned what your hands and mouths can say without words, grounded yourselves when anxiety knocked, played with senses and props, built desire all day long, and lingered in slow, seven-course lovemaking. You welcomed tools when they helped, pillows when they comforted, and each other every single time—and here you are at the end, but really at the beginning.

Your marriage bed is holy ground. It is where two image-bearers become one flesh, where covenant love becomes human, where the Song of Songs comes alive in your own story. It is where shame loses its grip, where pleasure is called good, where laughter and tears both belong, and where God Himself smiles at the delight of His children.

Keep coming back to these pages whenever you need a refresher, a laugh, or a gentle nudge. Keep talking. Keep touching. Keep praying together naked and unashamed. God wants your intimacy to thriving, playful, and deeply connected, mind, body, and soul.

OUR CLOSING PRAYER

Father, You are never in a hurry with us. Teach us to make love the way You love—lavishly, slowly, creatively, and with great joy. Let our bedroom be a place where shame has no address, and joy has an open invitation. Let our intimacy reflect Your fierce, tender, unbreakable covenant with us. Keep us curious about each other, quick to forgive, slow to criticize, and always eager to bless. We trust You with our hearts, our bodies, and our future. In the strong name of Jesus, amen.

Now go. Love well. Grow your connected intimacy.

Together, you are capable.

Together, you are strong.

Together, there is hope.

ACKNOWLEDGMENTS

When someone models something beautiful, it changes what you believe is possible.

To our youth pastors—Mitch and Melissa, and Stephen and Amber—thank you for showing us, long before we had the words for it, what a shame-free approach to marriage and intimacy actually looks like. You didn't just teach it. You lived it. That mattered more than you know.

ABOUT THE AUTHORS

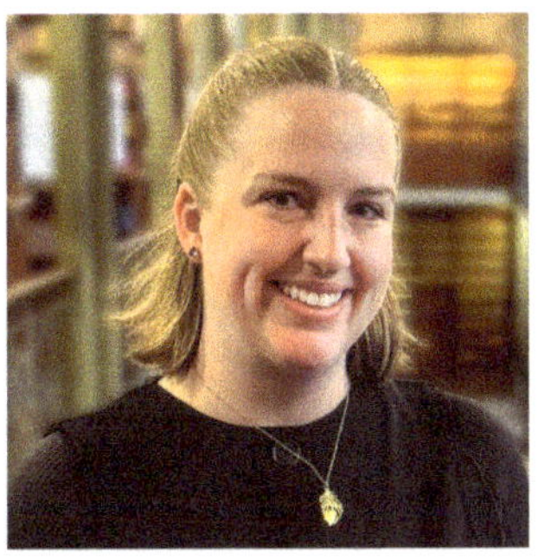

Kelsey Mathias, OTR/L, PRPC, is an occupational therapist and nationally recognized leader in maternal and pelvic health. She specializes in perinatal care, intimacy, and relationship well-being, bridging clinical science with real-life application for individuals, couples, and families. Kelsey is a co-creator and advisor of multiple national continuing education programs for pelvic health professionals and has contributed to large-scale clinical education initiatives across health care systems. She is also co-founder of Connected Intimacy, a platform dedicated to reframing conversations around intimacy with the goal of helping Christian couples have shame-free sex in mind, body, and soul.

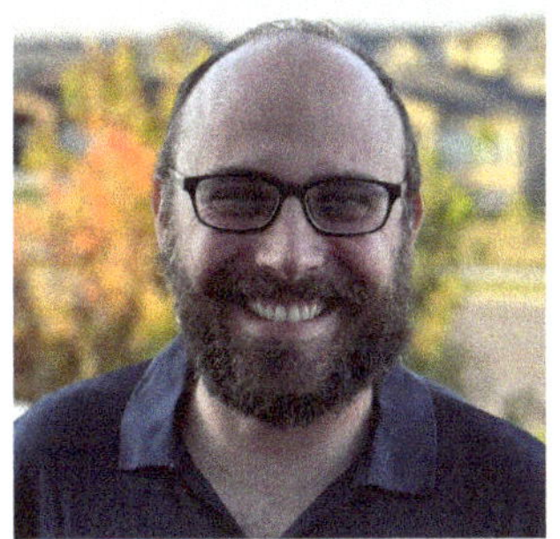

Larry Mathias is a pastor, community leader, and communicator with over a decade of experience in high-impact pastoral ministry. He specializes in organizational health, spiritual formation, and leadership development, and has served on leadership teams in churches of varying sizes to help individuals and families navigate faith, identity, and growth. With a background in digital design and multimedia storytelling, Larry bridges ancient truths with modern culture. He lives in Colorado Springs, where he continues to advocate for transparent, mission-driven communication that builds healthy, resilient communities. Larry is also co-founder of Connected Intimacy.